Oxford Guide to
Metaphors in CBT

Oxford Guides in Cognitive Behavioural Therapy

Oxford Guide to Low Intensity CBT Interventions
Bennett-Levy, Richards, Farrand, Christensen, Griffiths, Kavanagh, Klein, Lau, Proudfoot, Ritterband, Williams, and White

Oxford Guide to Surviving as a CBT Therapist
Mueller, Kennerley, McManus, and Westbrook

Oxford Guide to Metaphors in CBT
Stott, Mansell, Salkovskis, Lavender, and Cartwright-Hatton

Also Published by Oxford University Press

The Oxford Guide to Behavioural Experiments in Cognitive Therapy
Bennett-Levy, Butler, Fennell, Hackmann, Mueller, and Westbrook

Oxford Guide to Metaphors in CBT
Building Cognitive Bridges

Richard Stott
Warren Mansell
Paul Salkovskis
Anna Lavender
Sam Cartwright-Hatton

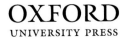

OXFORD
UNIVERSITY PRESS

OXFORD
UNIVERSITY PRESS

Great Clarendon Street, Oxford OX2 6DP

Oxford University Press is a department of the University of Oxford.
It furthers the University's objective of excellence in research, scholarship,
and education by publishing worldwide in

Oxford New York

Athens Auckland Bangkok Bogotá Buenos Aires Cape-Town
Chennai Dar es Salaam Delhi Florence Hong Kong Istanbul Karachi
Kolkata Kuala Lumpur Madrid Melbourne Mexico City Mumbai Nairobi
Paris São Paulo Shanghai Singapore Taipei Tokyo Toronto Warsaw

with associated companies in Berlin Ibadan

Oxford is a registered trade mark of Oxford University Press
in the UK and in certain other countries

Published in the United States
by Oxford University Press Inc., New York

© Oxford University Press, 2010

The moral rights of the author have been asserted

Database right Oxford University Press (maker)

First published 2010

All rights reserved. No part of this publication may be reproduced,
stored in a retrieval system, or transmitted, in any form or by any means,
without the prior permission in writing of Oxford University Press,
or as expressly permitted by law, or under terms agreed with the appropriate
reprographics rights organization. Enquiries concerning reproduction
outside the scope of the above should be sent to the Rights Department,
Oxford University Press, at the address above

You must not circulate this book in any other binding or cover
and you must impose this same condition on any acquirer

British Library Cataloguing in Publication Data

Data available

Library of Congress Cataloguing in Publication Data

Data available

Typeset in Minion by Glyph International, Bangalore, India
Printed in Great Britain
on acid-free paper by
MPG Books Group,
Bodmin and King's Lynn

ISBN 978–0–19–920749–7

10 9 8 7 6 5 4

Acknowledgements

In many respects it is impossible to adequately acknowledge all the people who have contributed to making this book possible. Since the inception of cognitive therapy, many therapy trainers have generously disseminated their clinical wisdom through successive generations of therapists. Metaphors have percolated through the therapy networks, often to be recycled, adapted, honed, and passed on once more. As with a traditional verse or great melody, the origin often gets lost and the metaphors get absorbed into therapy 'lore'.

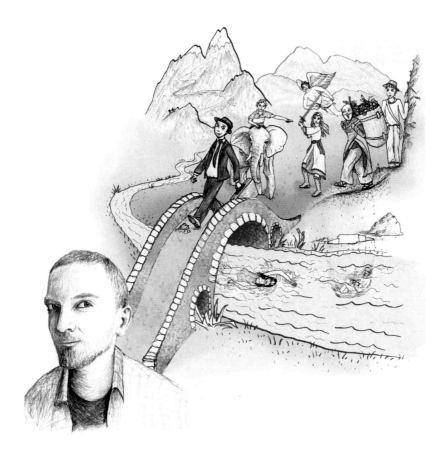

Nevertheless, there are many people whose contributions, both direct and indirect, we have valued enormously and would wish to acknowledge explicitly. Charlotte Turtle, our cartoonist, has successfully brought many of the metaphors in this book to life with her skilful artwork, for which we are extremely grateful. Metaphors bridge the verbal and imaginal, and without her imagery we feel this book would be fundamentally incomplete.

Many people enthusiastically shared a wealth of material, including Lorraine Bell, Aidan Bucknall, Jeremy Gauntlett-Gilbert, Sarah Goff, Nick Grey, Ian Lowens, Helen Morey, and Glenn Waller. We would also like to thank Sharif El-Leithy, Jon Wheatley, and Victoria Oldfield for their contributions and numerous discussions on both the theoretical and practical side of employing metaphor in CBT.

A few individuals also helped 'steer the conceptual ship' in the earlier stages of planning and developing this book. Particularly, we valued the insightful wisdom, input and encouragement of Gillian Butler, Ann Hackmann, and David M. Clark.

We are also conscious that some notable exponents of cognitive therapy have advocated metaphor and contributed much to this field, in workshops, lectures and in their writings. Paul Gilbert, Steven Hayes, Richard Kopp, Robert Leahy, Michael Otto, Christine Padesky, and Adrian Wells are certainly in this category. The writings of Paul Blenkiron are also much to be valued and welcomed.

We are most grateful to our editor Martin Baum, as well as Jennifer Lunsford, Gayathri Bellan and all the other staff at Oxford University Press and Glyph International who have worked hard with us over the past few months. In addition, huge thanks are owed to Sophie Wallace-Hadrill for her thorough and thoughtful proof-reading and comments.

Finally, we would wish to acknowledge the implicit help of many people from other therapy disciplines, psycholinguistics, and the field of communications, whose ideas have helped shape our own thinking in this complex and fertile area.

Foreword

Aaron T. Beck

Cognitive Therapy is a set of therapeutic interventions that aims to help patients learn to solve current problems and change dysfunctional thinking patterns that contribute to maladaptive emotions and behaviours. When I first started using the set of interventions that I later called "cognitive therapy" I theorized that disordered thinking lay at the heart of psychiatric disorders such as anxiety and depression. I observed that patients demonstrated systematic cognitive biases in the ways in which they interpreted aspects of their experience and that these cognitive biases played a significant role in the maladaptive emotions and behavioural responses they were currently struggling with. In my clinical work it became clear that working collaboratively with patients to identify and evaluate distorted or unhelpful thoughts and beliefs and adopt more adaptive ways of thinking and reacting was associated with an almost immediate reduction in the patient's symptoms. I also discovered that training clients in this process so that they could become their own "therapist" helped them to sustain these improvements even after they discontinued therapy.

The system of psychotherapy which I had begun based on these principles has since been empirically validated by myself and other investigators for a variety of psychiatric disorders. The interventions associated with this system of psychotherapy have evolved so that Cognitive Therapy (CT) today represents the blending of clinical art and science. *The Oxford Guide to Metaphors in CBT: Building Cognitive Bridges* is an excellent example of the evolution of CT. This book describes the theoretical and practical ways in which metaphor can be used to help patients transform the negative meanings which drive their problems in the "here and now" and are the source of so much suffering.

Early on in the development of CT, I noted the power of metaphor in the generation of and ability to sustain helpful alternative ways of thinking about and understanding the patient's world, often starting (as this book suggests) from the patients' own use of metaphor. For example, in my book entitled Cognitive Therapy for Depression (Beck et al. 1979), I described the usefulness of metaphor in my work with a depressed patient who had relapsed and was experiencing suicidal thoughts. Specifically, I reminded this patient that earlier in therapy she had said "I may feel like a mouse but I have the heart of a lion".

I pointed out that not only did the recollection of this metaphorical phrase recapture the attitude and feelings that she needed to continue her struggle against depression, but it also subtly gave her credit for persisting.

"The burglar example", one of the most widely used examples of metaphor in CT, also comes from the same book (Beck et al., 1979). For therapists and patients alike, this has been a simple but highly effective introduction to the principles of cognitive theory and how cognitive therapy helps people to change their perspectives on the problems they face. In this story, the patient is invited to think of someone asleep at home while alone in the house who hears a crash in another room. The patient is invited to consider what would likely be running through his mind, how that would impact his feelings, and the ways in which he would seek to protect himself (i.e. his behaviour). In the second story someone is asleep at home, hears the same noise but instead thinks "The windows have been left open and the wind has caused something to fall over". A primary aim of the discussion that follows with the client is to highlight how these alternative thoughts are associated with different and less negative feelings (e.g. annoyance that one of his kids left the window open instead of intense anxiety associated with thoughts that a burglar was in the house) and motivate a different behavioural response. The therapist could summarize the discussion by saying "Okay. Now, what this example shows us is that there are usually a number of ways in which you can interpret a situation. Also, the way in which you interpret the situation affects your feelings and behaviour".

Later in my career, I suggested that the use of metaphors can be helpful in allowing patients to reflect on their core beliefs "by reflecting on a different situation". For instance, guiding a patient who concluded that she must be "bad" because her mother ill-treated her as a child to reflect upon the story of Cinderella was a helpful way of reflecting on alternatives relating to the patient's past experience so that she could re-appraise her present experience (Beck et al., 1985).

Cognitive therapy seeks to harness the best of clinical art and science in the service of helping people to overcome the burden of maladaptive negative beliefs, biases in thinking and their emotional and behavioural consequences. This book manages to strike a perfect balance between the apparently conflicting demands of facilitating acceptance of the patient's experience and the need to allow them to consider alternative ways of thinking about their self, experience and future. The end result is a book that empowers patients to commit themselves to new ways of reacting to and interacting with the world so that they can gain control over their symptoms and live more fulfilling lives.

ATB

Contents

1 Introduction *1*

2 Historical roots, theory, and conceptualization *5*

3 Clinical use of metaphor *27*

4 Principles, format, and context of CBT *49*

5 Conceptualizing cognition and metacognition *75*

6 Depression *103*

7 Anxiety disorders *127*

8 Bipolar disorders and mood swings *159*

9 Psychosis *173*

10 Eating disorders *189*

11 Interpersonal difficulties *201*

12 Working with parents *215*

13 Clinical art and clinical science of metaphor in CBT: future directions *227*

References *237*

Index *245*

Chapter 1

Introduction

Overview

> Metaphors are such lovely, complete visual packages. They are so available and
> immediate. They can be the distillate of hours of therapeutic work.

> Margaret Hovanec, Academy of Cognitive Therapy Newsletter, April 2003

The business of cognitive therapy is to transform meanings. What better way
to achieve this than through a metaphor? It straddles two different domains at
once, providing a conceptual bridge from a problematic interpretation to a
fresh new perspective that can cast one's experiences in a new light. The use of
metaphors is considered by some to be an essential Rosetta Stone that links
different areas of thought and which is needed for the development of culture.
Metaphors are found across different languages and peppered throughout
most texts. We have squeezed at least six into the paragraph so far.

It is striking how the simplest metaphor can be used again and again with
different clients, yet still achieves its desired effect. One such example is the
"broken leg" metaphor for depression. Clients with depression are understandably frustrated with their symptoms. They may often push themselves to
get better or tell themselves that they *should* be better by now. As a therapist, it
is fair to ask, would the client be so harsh and demanding on herself after getting a broken leg? A broken leg needs time to heal and you need to begin to
walk on it gradually as it builds up in strength. "You can't run before you can
walk," and if you try, you are likely to make it worse. It is still surprising the
number of clients for whom this simple metaphor is enlightening—changing
their view of their symptoms as a sign of their own laziness and worthlessness
to a view of them as part of an understandable illness—that their condition,
while open to improvement, cannot get better overnight. It is tempting to suggest that metaphors of this kind should be part of our education, rather than
an idea that people stumble upon when reaching an impasse in their lives.

Over the years, we (the authors) have encountered (and in some cases generated) so many helpful metaphors during our clinical and academic encounters
with cognitive behaviour therapy (CBT) that we decided to try to draw many of
these gems together in one place. As we did so, we became increasingly aware

that metaphor and meaning are fundamentally intertwined, and that metaphor is an instinctive, often essential mechanism via which we comprehend and communicate our experiences. In the spirit of CBT we decided to make it a collaborative project, stretching our tentacles broadly so as to draw in contributions from a wide range of sources. We have scrutinized published work, contacted established clinicians who have written on the use of metaphors, made requests to jobbing clinicians and clinical researchers, and scoured around for the clearest examples of good practice. However, we did not wish simply to create a "directory" of metaphors, with no guidance offered as to how to employ them. Therefore, in our discussions with colleagues, we enquired extensively as to *how* people have used metaphor, as well as *what* those metaphors were. It is our view that metaphors in CBT achieve their most potent effect when skilfully embedded into the therapeutic conversation, and we wished to crystallize this wisdom in the book. For this reason, the chapters are complemented throughout with vignettes and therapeutic dialogues to illustrate the way that metaphors can be used effectively in CBT.

We have paid close attention to how to organize this book. Chapter 2 describes the historical roots, theory, and scientific background behind the use of metaphors in therapy. Chapter 3 is devoted to an overview of the clinical use of metaphors in CBT, including how to adapt client-generated metaphors. In Chapter 4, we start with the use of metaphors in explaining the principles and format of CBT, followed by a full chapter (Chapter 5) on metaphors that illustrate cognitive and metacognitive processes. While these early chapters utilize metaphors for any kind of presenting problem or population, Chapters 6 to 10 illustrate metaphors for specific presenting problems: depression, anxiety, bipolar disorders, psychosis, and eating disorders. Chapter 11 is devoted to understanding interpersonal difficulties and life span development using metaphor and Chapter 12 explains the colourful use of metaphor in CBT that may be used for parents of anxious or depressed children. Finally, in Chapter 13, we offer some suggestions for future directions in clinical practice and research in the area of metaphor in CBT. A comprehensive index should also assist in navigating to the most relevant sections. We hope that the book can either be read from start to finish (if you really have that much time in your busy clinical schedule), or alternatively can be dipped into, as and when relevant.

Many of the metaphors in this book are accompanied by memorable cartoons, thanks to the artistic work of Charlotte Turtle. In some cases, these may act as a pictorial "aide memoire" for you, the reader, in lodging a metaphor in your mind. In other cases, you may consider that a copy of the cartoon would be helpful for your clients, as an adjunct to a relevant part of your therapy.

You are warmly encouraged to make use of them in this way. Alternatively, you may find they act as a stimulus for imagination, perhaps inspiring a variant of the metaphor in the minds of client and/or therapist. People picture scenes in different ways, and each cartoon represents just one possible interpretation of the metaphorical theme in question. However you choose to view or use them, we trust they will be valuable.

What are the aims of this book?

Increasingly, CBT therapists have become interested in using metaphors. In recent years, metaphors have formed the subject of academic papers, clinical workshops, and conference symposia. We believed that there was a role for a book with three aims in mind:

1. *Clinical practice:* to crystallize the most effective ways to utilize metaphors in CBT and help generate new effective metaphors
2. *Theory and research:* to review the scientific foundations for the use of metaphor and to foster an empirical approach to their use in CBT
3. *Reference:* to utilize metaphors throughout the text to illustrate their use in clinical practice and provide them as a resource for therapists.

We are well aware that none of these aims are fully achievable in one book, but they have provided a standard to aim for and pursue in later work. This book is more than a resource for clinicians to use as a "cookbook" approach to selecting the most relevant metaphors; its aim is to lay the theoretical, practical, and empirical foundations for the effective use of metaphors, within the collaborative and empirical spirit of CBT.

What is included? The wider concept of a metaphor

A metaphor literally means "a figure of speech in which an expression is used to refer to something that it does not literally denote in order to suggest a similarity." Some of the examples of metaphors are "The world's a stage," "he was a lion in battle," "drowning in debt," and "a sea of troubles." In CBT we may use simple figures of speech in this way (e.g. "try to ride the wave of anxiety") but often the metaphors are more elaborate visual descriptions that can resemble short stories and parables. These well-developed narrative metaphors seem, at least on the surface, to have more clinical utility. Similarly, poems, scenes from books, plays and films, works of art, and news stories have the capacity to transform meaning by sharing a conceptual similarity to our client's experiences, yet superficially involving very different subject matter. Therefore we have included each of these within our wider concept of a metaphor.

We also consider analogies and similes under the umbrella term "metaphor" for the sake of simplicity.

We hope that you find this book valuable in your practice of CBT and as stimulating to read as we found to write. The creativity of metaphor is one of the aspects of therapy that we thrive on, and so please join us as we build cognitive bridges and encourage you and your clients to do the same.

Chapter 2

Historical roots, theory, and conceptualization

Introduction

A basic premise of the cognitive model is that people in psychological distress view their world through a distorting lens. Some thoughts and perceptions are interpreted according to a person's own idiosyncratic rules and "filters," and such people change their behaviour accordingly. Processes of this kind can make warm and sociable people feel unwanted, reasonable and fair people feel guilty, normal people feel they stand out from the crowd, and thin people feel fat. Typically, however, such a distorting lens is *not* universally applied across other great swathes of cognition. In striking contrast, such individuals often maintain a highly robust grip upon most of their fundamental conceptual world, including the nature of up and down, of day and night, the fact that journeys have a beginning and an end, the fact that trees grow upward, branch, and need water, the fact that buildings need foundations, and so on. Helping people in distress to use metaphor to bring their accurate understanding of the fundamentals of their experience to bear on areas of distortion is not only possible but desirable, as the new understanding is firmly founded in undistorted reality and therefore is particularly likely to be sustained. The aim of this chapter is to introduce the concept of metaphor, survey its historical journey as a linguistic device and a cognitive construct, and introduce a rationale for using metaphor to provide a powerful therapeutic bridge between these disparate domains of distress and of grounded reality.

Metaphor is traditionally defined as a figure of speech that implies comparison between two unlike entities, e.g. *All the world's a stage, all the men and women merely players* (Shakespeare). A closely related linguistic form is that of the simile, where the comparison is made explicit, i.e. *Her creative ideas were like a breath of fresh air*. We certainly do not have to search long to discover evidence of metaphor throughout much ordinary dialogue. Consider how frequently one hears the following metaphorical expressions, when people speak of their own concerns:

I want to *move on* and *put this behind* me.
I feel completely *trapped* [solutions as exit routes].

I don't know how much more *I can take* [stress as a burden / causing injury].
These issues are very *deep-rooted*.
I think one day I'm going to just *snap*.
I feel like there's a *dark cloud hanging over me*.
There must be a *way through this* [problems as physical obstructions].
Deep down I'm not sure what I really want.

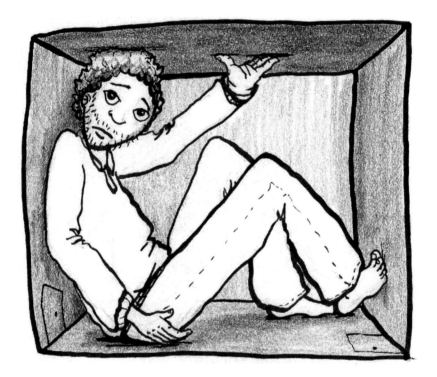

Metaphor typically acts as a bridge between a source domain, which is more concrete or more familiar, and a target domain, which is more abstract or less familiar. For cognitive therapists, this should be priceless, as those in psychological distress are often trying to wrestle with abstract concepts, such as different kinds of thinking processes, or behaviours that may be counterproductive despite their initial appeal.

One client recently used a metaphor during therapy to summarize her feelings to one of us. She said that she had spent her life running as fast as she could up an escalator, but unfortunately it was a "down" escalator. She was becoming tired and going nowhere. In this way the client had vividly and concretely encapsulated a whole range of related ideas: an abstract sense of struggle, a motivation to change held back by feelings of lack of agency, a frustration at a system seemingly designed to thwart her efforts, the inability to further her own goals, and the feeling of loss of hope. Later in the chapter we will examine more closely the theory underpinning effective metaphor use in cognitive therapy. First, however, we should place metaphor in its historical context.

A brief history of metaphor

The metaphor is not a recent linguistic phenomenon. An anonymous Egyptian poem from circa 2000 BC contemplates death as follows:

> Death is before me today
> Like the sky when it clears
> Like a man's wish to see home after numberless years of captivity.

> (W.S. Merwin, trans. 1968)

Indeed, there is an argument that the core cognitive processes mediating metaphor have roots far back in our evolutionary history. It has been proposed, for example, that some higher-order apes successfully process concept relationships of the form "A is to B as C is to D." Gillan, Premack and Woodruff (1981) found that their chimpanzee Sarah could successfully identify the missing piece of such a puzzle from a selection, when three of the four elements were presented. This was found both with abstract geometric shapes, for example, coloured triangles and crescent shapes, and objects functionally related, for example, a key, a padlock, a can-opener, and a can. More recent research has suggested that this particular chimpanzee could construct, as well as solve, these forms of analogical relationships (Oden, Thompson, & Premack, 2001).

The telling of wise tales

Metaphor, when extended into a brief coherent story, can deliver succinct implicit messages typically to convey abstract principles. Cultural wisdom, moral values, and lessons of life have long been embedded in and imparted through fictional narrative, such as the parables of Jesus, the tales of the legendary Mullah Nasruddin, myths, legends, and the many and various fables and fairy stories that enthrall generations of children. In many cases, this form has an agenda—there is a message which is designed to be imparted, the meaning of which is found some way beneath the surface of the story itself. Sometimes, the meaning or lesson may be summarized explicitly for the listener at the end, with the aid of a pithy maxim. In other cases, the story is left to ferment in the mind of the listener, with the hope that the onward connections to real life get made, consciously or unconsciously. The fictional component of such tales is packaging, but arguably essential. For example, the brief diversion into another character's life may permit sufficient engagement and attention, and attain sufficient vividness that the message becomes persuasive and enduring.

In addition, the fictional narrative allows a balance to be struck between obtaining a useful distance from oneself and yet also achieving a resonance with one's own issues and experiences. This may further optimize the power of the message and add to the compelling nature of the wise tale. The metaphor helpfully provides the vehicle that allows more rapid conceptual travel than would otherwise be the case.

Figurative language

Nonliteral or figurative use of language is widespread in literature and has been an almost defining characteristic of poetry through the ages. Poets have exploited the capacity of language to go beyond a direct communication of meaning and to evoke aesthetic sensory responses in the listener. They manage to do this partly through acoustic and rhythmic devices. Yet, importantly, they use the "metaphorical juxtaposition" of disparate ideas, and the blending of fragments of meaning to render a "gestalt," which transcends the individual words or ideas taken in isolation (we will discuss later how this might happen from a psychological perspective). Indeed, "what the poem means" is sometimes not the point, as articulated by Archibald MacLeish in the final lines of his poem "Ars Poetica": *A poem should not mean, but be.* Sometimes, metaphorical comparison is stated explicitly, as in Shakespeare's celebrated Sonnet 18, *Shall I compare thee to a summer's day?* Other times, the blending is done implicitly (e.g. *the slings and arrows of outrageous fortune*). The notion that, without explicit meaning or classic syntax, words themselves carry rich connotation and evoke complex sensory imagery, was a theme espoused by the writer and poet Gertrude Stein in the early twentieth century. Her famous line *A rose is a rose is a rose* encapsulates the idea that the word "rose" itself evokes the sweet smell, the red colour, and in essence, makes the rose "come alive," without the need to spell it out or describe it. In fact, she suggested, slightly boastfully perhaps, that her line had made a rose red for the first time in a hundred years of poetry! (Stein, 1947).

Philosophical scepticism

However, metaphor has not always been popular among great thinkers and scientists through the ages. Aristotle believed that mastery of metaphor was a sign of linguistic genius, but thought it too ornamental for scientific or philosophical use. It has been dismissed by others as flowery, superficial, or deviant from ordinary literal language, and at worst representing fuzzy, vague, or lazy-minded thinking. Such language might belong in the domain of the poet, perhaps, but certainly not in that of the serious thinker or hard-nosed scientist dealing with precise truths or hypotheses. This view of metaphorical language became especially prevalent during the period of the Enlightenment in the eighteenth century, when human reason and rationality were seen as superior and as essential elements in combating ignorance and building a better world. The British philosopher John Locke, in 1690, had the following to say about figurative language:

> if we would speak of things as they are, we must allow that all the art of rhetoric, besides order and clearness; all the artificial and figurative application of words eloquence hath invented, are for nothing else but to insinuate wrong ideas, move the passions, and thereby mislead the judgement; and so indeed are perfect cheats. And therefore, however laudable or allowable oratory may render them in harangues and popular addresses, they are certainly, in all discourses that pretend to inform or instruct, wholly to be avoided.
>
> (Locke, 1979)

Locke, in common with other thinkers of his time, clearly believed that inform-ative language should "tell it how it is." Ironically, perhaps, one of the ideas for which he is most famous is how children are born into the world with no innate knowledge or mental content, his so-called *tabula rasa* (blank slate). Locke's *tabula rasa* proved to be an enduring and highly influential metaphor of mind.

Political and rhetorical use of metaphor

With or without the approval of scientists and philosophers, the powerful per-suasive potential of metaphorical expression has been fully exploited by rulers and politicians throughout the ages. Winston Churchill spoke memorably about the "iron curtain descending across Europe" and "the gathering storm" as a metaphor for the threats to peace in the interwar years. Martin Luther King, champion of American civil rights, on the day before he was killed in 1968, famously spoke of the mountain-top over which he had looked, and seen into the "promised land."

There have been a few scientific attempts to analyze political metaphor in a controlled setting. Bosman (1987) experimentally investigated the persuasive effects of political metaphors upon participants' attitudes towards a political party. It was found that not only did metaphor systematically affect attitudes, but the specific persuasive effects of each metaphor depended upon the politi-cal party to which they were applied. Bosman inferred that metaphors operate as a persuasive device not merely by their emotional power but by the cognitive structuring of the domain concept in the mind of the observer.

Perhaps unsurprisingly, therefore, some have also sought to cast metaphor in the role of manipulative language—a central weapon in the politician's armory of persuasive rhetoric and spin, often underhand, misleading, or even plain dishonest. There is certainly no doubt that politicians, and those seeking to change the minds of others, have something of a love affair with this form of figurative language. Just consider the impact of the phrases "rivers of blood," "sword of truth," and "war on terror." Such examples are vivid, dramatic, highly memorable, and, for better or worse, highly influential. In many cases the enduring metaphor may even outlive the identity of its master.

Constructivist view

The implied, dichotomous distinction between literal and metaphorical language has been referred to as the "double language thesis" (Beardsley, 1972). However, this distinction has been challenged in recent times. Indeed, the movement known as constructivism brought a fresh perspective to the nature of all linguistic activity. Within this framework, all language is regarded, to a greater or lesser extent, as being a creative and generative activity, and is in the active business of constructing meaning. For example, the statement *I used all my skills to conquer the problems I faced* is relatively literal and would not obviously reside in the domain of poetry or "ornamental" language. Nevertheless, the single word "conquer" introduces meaning from the domain of battle, and thereby constructs a wealth of associated meaning and implication as to how the problems were viewed (as an enemy or threat), and the resultant outcome (triumph, high esteem, problems defeated). Indeed, the word "wealth" in that last sentence also imported meaning from another domain, implying a sense of quality, quantity, and richness. In fact, metaphorical activity seems to be alive and well virtually wherever you look. The constructivist view argues that literal and overtly "metaphorical" language lie along a continuum, varying only in the degree and explicitness of their generation of new meaning.

Metaphor brings together two distinct domains of knowledge and meaning. Within the constructivist, generative view of language, then, metaphor can go far beyond a mere "interesting comparison" between the two domains; rather it actually cross-fertilizes meaning. Ivor Richards, one of the founders of modern literary criticism, articulated this "interactive" view of metaphor in his influential book *The Philosophy of Rhetoric* (Richards, 1936). He regarded the resultant metaphorical meaning as transcending the meaning of both the original conceptual structures. This is a far cry from a view of metaphor as linguistic frills, or icing on cakes. Metaphor has the potential to operate at the forefront of the meaning-construction industry.

Lakoff and Johnson's conceptual metaphors

A highly influential account of metaphor has come from the work of cognitive linguists Lakoff and Johnson (1980) with their "conceptual metaphor" framework. They proposed that metaphor is a fundamental property of concepts, moulding our very thinking, and understanding and not just a feature of language. To take one example, they suggest a key conceptual metaphor we hold is "LIFE IS A JOURNEY." They would argue that substantial linguistic evidence points to our concept of life (the *target domain*) being shaped by that of our concept of a journey (the *source domain*). Expressions such as "I am moving on in life," "I am reaching the end of my life," "I don't ever look back," "The years seem to pass so quickly" etc. might attest to this. Indeed, it may be that life is too abstract a concept to grapple with mentally without pinning it to the more concrete notion of the journey. Lakoff and Johnson's thesis is that our mental representations of complex concepts are inherently structured by a set of metaphorical correspondences, which give rise to our cognitive processing of those concepts. In addition, these underlying conceptual configurations allow us to generate a surface stream of metaphorical linguistic expressions and also to comprehend figurative language spoken or written by others.

Lakoff and his colleagues have amassed and attempted to classify a huge assortment of conceptual metaphors, which they believe configure our understanding of complex and abstract concepts including love, life, anger, theories, causality, and the nature of the mind. As Kövecses (2002) describes, many of the *source* domains drawn upon in conceptual metaphor are relatively concrete and familiar, including the human body, health and illness, animals, plants, buildings, machines and tools, games, money, food, hot and cold, light and darkness, forces, movement, and direction. Table 2.1 illustrates a few examples of common conceptual metaphors and the expressions to which they give rise.

Lakoff and Johnson's conceptual metaphors have immediate appeal, and offer a plausible account of the human mind's ready ability both to produce and comprehend novel metaphoric utterances, which have been hung upon the putative underlying conceptual structure. The enormous influence of this approach is seen in its uptake across multiple discliplines, including politics (Bosman, 1987; Paris, 2002), war studies (Lule, 2004), and religion (Soskice, 1987). Nevertheless, there have been several critics of the theory. McGlone (2007) argues, for example, that cognitive structures underpinning abstract concepts (e.g. theories) cannot literally be subsumed by the cognitive structure of, say, buildings—we know very clearly that theories are not actually buildings. The real nature and extent of these alleged conceptual correspondences should be subjected to more rigorous empirical test, and not merely inferred from the plethora of surface-level idioms found in everyday discourse, according to McGlone (2007). Others have argued that there is considerably more fluidity to the nature of cognitive processing that underlies metaphor use and comprehension. For example, a novel metaphor may be processed more as a literal comparison, and a conventional metaphor more at the level of categorization

Table 2.1 Some examples of common conceptual metaphors and associated metaphorical expressions

Underlying conceptual metaphor	Example expressions to which it gives rise
Theories are buildings	I need to *construct* a strong argument That theory sounds rather *shaky* What is that idea *founded upon?*
Argument is war	He *attacked* every point I made You need to *defend* your position strongly I think we are *winning* the argument
Anger is hot fluid in a container	She was *boiling* with rage I think he's going to *blow* a gasket I can feel *my temperature* rising but I'm trying to *keep* a lid on it
Complex abstract systems are plants	There are many *branches* of the organisation This endeavour is *bearing fruit* at last You will encounter *deep-rooted* traditions
Time is motion	The due date has *passed.* They are three hours *behind.* With the *passage* of time it will become a more *distant* memory.

(Bowdle & Gentner, 2005). Nevertheless, Lakoff and Johnson's identification of many clusters of apparently consistent mappings between abstract and concrete concepts, and the realization that our language and thought about many abstract ideas is fundamentally anchored to other domains of cognition, was an important and major step forward.

Metaphor in therapy

The fact that metaphor has long been used to manipulate minds has not precluded its judicious and benevolent use. Indeed, metaphor has a significant tradition in certain therapeutic approaches. One notable advocate was the influential American psychiatrist and "father of clinical hypnosis" Milton Erickson. Erickson made an art out of incorporating metaphor and personal stories into his therapeutic work (e.g. Rosen, 1982). By telling metaphorical tales, Erickson was, in many respects, following the ancient communicative traditions of parable and fable. His aim, particularly, was to activate meaning in his clients at an implicit or subliminal level. For example, he might share an anecdote with his client that, while overtly representing a story of difficulty or struggle, covertly implied an association between struggle and strength. In this way, a reconfiguration of meaning associations was believed to occur in the client's unconscious mind. His work inspired a number of other branches of therapy, including Bandler and Grinder's neurolinguistic programming (NLP) and others (e.g. Gordon, 1978; Burns, 2001). His influence upon the use of metaphor in family therapy has also been significant (e.g. Lankton & Lankton, 1989).

Psychoanalytic traditions also embrace metaphor extensively. Much of the interpretative approach rests on the assumption that the accessible parts of thought, speech, and experience (not least dreams, and the well-known "Freudian slips") may represent a disguised, masked form of the underlying unconscious conflicts—the unconscious thus reveals itself in symbols and metaphors (Bettleheim, 1984). In some cases, even when a client believes their stream of thinking is quite literal, the psychoanalytic practitioner may suspect a metaphorical meaning. For example, a dream of having a car crash, or an illogical health anxiety about a skin condition, may be explored as metaphorical representations of unspoken anxieties from another part of the client's life.

Acceptance and commitment therapy (ACT) is another branch of therapy that makes rich use of metaphor. Having evolved from radical behaviourism, its theoretical underpinnings are grounded in a complex theory of human language and cognition, known as relational frame theory (RFT; Hayes, Barnes-Holmes, & Roche, 2001). This theory is a bold attempt to bring "verbal behaviour" back within the realm of behavioural analysis, although a full description is outside the scope of the present book. Metaphor, according to RFT, assists in transforming the "functions" (i.e. effects) of the stimuli in question. For example, the phrase "cats are dictators" establishes a framework of coordination between cats and dictators, with the shared feature of "demandingness." The relational network has been elaborated and the function of "cats" has been transformed.

From an ACT perspective, which sets great store by its pragmatic stance, use of metaphors in therapy is also seen as particularly powerful because it is not literal language; indeed they are often stories with a strong pictorial element. For example, ACT therapists might employ a "bad cup" metaphor to expose the linguistic confusion of evaluation versus description statements. Adjectives such as "good" and "bad" can masquerade as descriptions, whereas in reality "a good cup" only has meaning by virtue of a relationship to a person with opinions. This is in contrast to "a ceramic cup," which would maintain its validity even in the event of the death of all living creatures. A brief story and exploration about a bad cup serves as a metaphor to highlight what is otherwise an abstract philosophical idea. Overall, in ACT, metaphors are seen as establishing a setting in which overreliance on rationality is questioned, and which are also memorable and often applicable across many settings (Hayes, Stosahl, & Wilson, 1999).

Kopp (1995) has also advocated the use of metaphor in therapy and, in this case, not specifically allied to any particular therapeutic orientation. His approach is to assist the client in exploring and transforming their own meta-phors. First, a client is encouraged to explore and elaborate their metaphorical image. This is done by questions such as *When you say X [metaphor], what pictures come to mind?, If I were seeing it, what would I see?, What else is going on in the image?* and so on. Then a metaphoric transformation is invited, either with or without any prompts of content from the therapist (e.g. *If you could change the image in any way, how would you change it?*) Finally the client is invited to step back from the metaphor, and explore parallels between their metaphor and the original situation, including any implications of the trans-formation. Kopp's approach rests on the notion that metaphor is a distinct form of cognition, which unites the logical and imaginal—"metaphoric cognition"—and although this strong claim may not be fully substantiated, his ideas have considerable overlap and similarity with other therapeutic strate-gies, notably imagery rescripting (e.g. Smucker & Dancu, 1999). The metaphor work thus centres around a visual image, with any transformations closely tied to their meanings at a verbal, propositional level.

Rationale for metaphor use in cognitive therapy

Cognitive therapy has, as a central task, the aim of transforming meaning to further the client's goals and help journey towards a more helpful, realistic and adaptive view of the self and the world. Metaphor should therefore be a powerful companion.

Consider the scenario in which a therapist wishes to convey to a client with low self-esteem the idea that they may be employing selective attention to other people's comments about them, thereby deriving and committing to memory a biased and unhelpful view of themselves. The therapist enquires whether the client might be seeing things at present through a "gloomy pair of spectacles" (see also Chapter 6, p. 115). This simple and succinct metaphorical maneuver has a variety of effects. First, it activates an intact conceptual struc-ture in the client as to what happens when tinted spectacles are worn—the world changes colour and no longer looks quite real. Second, therefore, another important cognitive structure is activated, the understanding that perception and reality can be divergent, knowledge which may be only latently held by the client. Third, it implies a nonpermanence of the predicament; the tinted glasses can be removed. Fourth, it activates a mental model, which is nonblaming, i.e. the problem is with the spectacles, not with the client, and indeed the client can take responsibility for removing those spectacles and thereby seeing things in a different way. Fifth, a vivid image is created, succinctly crystallizing this new metaperspective, facilitating speedy recall and providing a convenient therapeutic hook upon which to hang a piece of therapeutic work and/or homework.

This example also perhaps illustrates three more general hypotheses, not mutually exclusive, which have emerged in the literature for understanding why people use metaphor so readily (Ortony, 1993). First is the inexpressibility hypothesis, which proposes that certain concepts are particularly problematic to express without recourse to metaphorical language. Second is the compactness hypothesis, which suggests that metaphor provides an efficient means to communicate, in a relatively small number of words, a rich and complex configuration of information structure, which literal language would not permit. Third is the vividness hypothesis, namely that metaphor can help a speaker or writer communicate the vividness of their phenomenological experience. To analyze these functions more closely, one might examine the domain of emotion, central to cognitive therapy. Indeed, emotion is an almost prototypical example of an abstract concept requiring use of a language for its analysis. However it is exceedingly difficult to capture the phenomenology of emotions without recourse to metaphor. Instead, we say "My blood was boiling," "He's feeling down," "She's on cloud nine," "I've been swept off my feet," "He's drowning his sorrows," "She wanted the ground to swallow her up," and so on. Kövecses (2000) argues how such metaphorical depictions of emotion are central to a more complete understanding of the complex experience of emotion, from a cognitive, social, cultural, and bodily perspective.

Another example illustrates how these three features of metaphor may also be of great value in cognitive therapy in the specific domain of formulation. Indeed, some components of formulation are inherently abstract, and yet need to provide the basis for implied therapeutic intervention. For example, in treatment of posttraumatic stress disorder (PTSD), it is useful to provide a basic formulation of the involuntary re-experiencing phenomenon, with an additional implication as to the therapeutic strategy required to "process" the troubling memory. One metaphor sometimes employed here is that of the oversized duvet (representing the traumatic memory) stuffed hurriedly into the usually organized linen cupboard, and the door slammed shut (see also Chapter 5, p. 85 and Chapter 7, p. 151). The door inevitably opens and the duvet falls out, motivating a cyclical process of stuffing it in and attempting to slam the door once more. The implication, to be elucidated with the client, is that a resolution is to be found only by removing the duvet, spending some time processing (folding) it and finally putting it away. In a compact and vivid way, this metaphor captures the inherently abstract notion of the traumatic re-experiencing phenomenon, and moreover provides a naturally implied link to the treatment strategy (reliving) required to address the problem. This is of particular benefit in PTSD as the reliving protocol can often be an aversive procedure and one which can otherwise be difficult to sell.

Within cognitive therapy, there are other compelling reasons to utilize metaphor. One is the powerful mnemonic capacity of metaphor. Most therapists would be familiar with the therapeutic problem of important material being forgotten, especially between sessions. Metaphors, however, often utilize rich and distinctive imagery, which is likely to be much more resilient to forgetting. For example, a discussion about the detrimental effect of safety behaviours, utilizing the image of the long-suffering builder's apprentice trying to hold up a wall (see Chapter 7, p. 137) is likely to result in better recall of the central message concerning safety behaviours, compared with a purely abstract discussion alone. Furthermore, such metaphors may become a shared reference point, allowing client and therapist to "speak the same language," which may enhance the feeling of being understood in the client and thus enhance the therapeutic bond. Importantly, also, judicious humour may be incorporated into the therapeutic dialogue in a manner which is supportive and allows the client to gently laugh at themselves in a sympathetic and constructive way. This theme is taken up further in the next chapter.

Types of metaphor in cognitive therapy

In the dialogue of therapy, metaphor can take on various forms. At one end of the spectrum, there may be expressions that are technically metaphorical but whose metaphorical character has been all but forgotten, sometimes dubbed "dead metaphors," e.g. *I've grasped what you are saying.* Then there are commonplace metaphorical expressions where the analogy may usefully be pictured and addressed, e.g. *I'm wrestling with this illness [Illness Is A Battle].* Then there are more elaborated and individualistic turns of phrase or scenario, e.g. *For the ten years of my marriage I was essentially trapped in a prison cell.* And then there are mini-anecdotes or analogous scenarios, which may be more elaborated and may contain a richer dramatic content and contextualization, allowing the imagination of client and therapist jointly to construct a scenario with its own internal logic, providing by analogy a new way of thinking about an old problem. Chapter 3 will examine more closely the practice of metaphor use in cognitive therapy.

An explicit approach

Unlike some other therapeutic approaches, the practice of cognitive therapy is founded upon an explicit and collaborative partnership between therapist and client, and in this book we follow Muran and DiGiuseppe (1990) in advocating an explicit approach to therapeutic utilization of metaphor. We can collaborate with our clients on the excursion through and incorporation of another meaning system, discuss the analogies being drawn, and obtain feedback on the fit, understanding and usefulness of any metaphor employed. Together we can suspend disbelief and picture progress in therapy as a hill climb with peaks and drops, or imagine our destructive eating patterns as an impossible form of breathing (see p. 195). This explicit approach in no way reduces the impact of new implicit associations being formed or strengthened; rather it keeps the whole process "on the table," providing for the client a valuable sense of ownership over their own changing perspectives. In addition it opens up the metaphor to intellectual scrutiny and refinement, helping to circumvent any misunderstandings or semantic mismatches between the client and the therapist.

Conceptual frameworks for meaning and metaphor

The aim of this section is to help shift from a basic rationale for why to use metaphors in cognitive therapy, to the conceptual underpinnings for how to do so. The conceptual framework we use builds on Lakoff and Johnson's earlier work, and resonates with the discussions of metaphor within literature and philosophy that we covered earlier. It also draws on contemporary work in psychology, cognitive neuroscience, and artificial intelligence. The essential premise is that metaphors allow us to use familiar sensory and motor experiences to understand, utilize, and modify more abstract concepts.

Metaphors as embodied cognition: a consensus of experts?

There appears to be an emerging consensus on how to conceptualize metaphors that builds upon the view the metaphors are a fundamental feature of human thought. In essence, a range of accounts converge on the view that metaphors are examples of embodied cognition. The terminology varies between accounts. We have already noted that within the field of cognitive linguistics, Lakoff and Johnson (1980) suggest that metaphors are based on meanings that are grounded in experience. They have termed these as *complex experiential gestalts*. Within neuroscience, the term *embodied experience* or *embodied meaning* is used (Feldman & Narayanan, 2004; Gibbs, 2003). These authors also suggest that the lived experience of sensorimotor co-ordination in the world is essential to establish embodied meanings. Within the field of artificial intelligence and computational mathematics, it has been proposed that metaphors depend on first-person agent environment coupling (Nehaniv, 1999). Finally, from a therapeutic perspective, Teasdale (1993) proposes that metaphor is tied to implicational, holistic meaning based on information from sensory and proprioceptive systems of the body.

It would probably be helpful to "put some flesh on the bones" at this stage, as these various terms can be quite confusing. One example is the use of the word "grasp" (Feldman & Narayanan, 2004). We grasp physical objects, but we also talk about grasping ideas. The sensorimotor processes involved in grasping are relatively well understood; the consensual view is that this first person experience of grasping through all of the sensorimotor machinery involved within the individual is an essential basis for establishing the meaning for the word "grasp," when used to apply to grasping ideas. It is generally thought that at either an implicit or explicit level, these processes are engaged in order to understand "grasping an idea." In other words, metaphors are dependent on their experiential basis, and this basis is complex and based on a history of interaction with the environment.

The purpose of metaphor use

There appears to be less written on what purpose metaphors serve. It seems implicit in many of the above accounts that metaphors promote the understanding of previously poorly understood domains. If we extend this to the clinical arena, then one would consider that metaphors help in the understanding of a presenting problem through links to embodied meaning within other domains—the depressed sportswoman is helped to understand graded increase in activity through her experience of training for a marathon—for example. There appears to be little consideration in the literature of what would make a person *want* to understand their problems better through metaphors. Presumably, the goal of wanting to understand one's problems (rather than ignoring or suppressing them) is a necessary condition before a metaphor can be used in therapy. It is an area that would be interesting to explore in future frameworks.

The process of metaphor use

Exactly how the process of using metaphors occurs is also unclear. Lakoff and Johnson (1980) propose that understanding a metaphor involves being able to superimpose the multidimensional structure of part of one concept upon the corresponding structural dimensions of a second concept. For example, "argument is war" is understood through matching components—turn taking as alternating attacks; leading the conversation as taking ground, etc. We would imagine that this process of superimposition would need to be "worked through" in consciousness when this metaphor is first encountered rather than happening instantaneously. Thus, returning to the earlier account, the process of forging a metaphor involves a concurrent awareness of matching components of the two concepts, *simulated as if embodied*, within the individual. Thus, a person who is asked whether arguments are like war for the first time would actually imagine a tirade of speech and a tatter of machine gun in their mind's eye, or another pairing of components between the two concepts. If this is that case, it provides certain clues as to other psychological components that are associated with metaphor use.

What components of cognition might metaphors involve?

1. *Awareness of imagery.* One clear conclusion from this conceptual approach to metaphors is that mental imagery as a simulation of embodied experience is necessary to understand metaphors. With this understanding comes the potential to grasp another domain of knowledge, which may help in resolving a personal problem. And so, attempts by the therapist to help the client to become aware of their own experience and their memories or simulations of that experience would be likely to help them to use metaphors effectively.

2. *Integration of verbal and imaginal.* Kopp (1995) explains how working on metaphors in therapy promotes the integration between verbal and imaginal cognition. There is evidence within the CBT literature that a preponderance of verbal processing in the form of rumination is associated with a range of psychological symptoms, overgeneral memory, and poor problem-solving (e.g. Watkins, 2008). Conversely, the ability to flexibly integrate verbal and sensory/perceptual information may be the hallmark of more adaptive processing.

3. *Holding two concepts in mind.* The ability to hold more than one thought in awareness at any one time may promote effective problem-solving through a wider consideration of the aspects of any problem—in order to link them, differentiate between them, or contrast them in some way.

4. *Awareness of commonalities despite superficial differences.* The process of metaphor use according to Lakoff and Johnson (1980) involves noticing similarities between two aspects of current cognition despite the superficial differences between them. There are reasons to think that this would be a highly adaptive cognitive skill, irrespective of whether a metaphor is the current content of awareness. Where this process leads commonalities

to become apparent, it would presumably enable adaptive experience gained in one domain to be applied to another within problem-solving. Speculatively, it is also possible that if people were to apply this process to their mental experience, they would come to realize that their own distressing experiences may be shared by other people, despite their superficial differences—a skill that helps the individual to realize that the facets of their own problem that might be shared with other people.

5. *Flexible use of multiple meanings.* A further interesting angle provided by Lakoff and Johnson (1980) is that having only one metaphor for a concept can be a limitation. Every metaphorical understanding of a concept highlights some aspects of its meaning at the expense of others. For example, understanding recovery from depression as preparing for a marathon effectively gets across that the process is gradual and purposeful, but ignores the likelihood that in recovery from depression it is often difficult to know what to do, in contrast to a marathon. Lakoff and Johnson propose that it is often more useful to have multiple metaphors for a concept than one, even if these multiple metaphors are inconsistent with one another. Thus, having the metaphor of recovery from depression as a marathon *and* as a "journey in the dark" is more helpful than having one alone. Thus, while it is helpful to have a more accurate metaphor, it can also be particularly useful to flexibly alternate between metaphors that capture different facets of a concept. Clinically, while care must be taken not to obscure or confuse by being overly complex, the use of multiple metaphors can also send a useful "meta-message": that there are different ways of looking at things.

A working theoretical model of metaphor use in cognitive therapy

The elements so far discussed can be summarized in a working theoretical model, depicted in Figure 2.1. Essentially there is a fourfold process of *activation, elaboration, synthesis,* and *reframe.* Specifically, by invoking a metaphor, two cognitive structures will be activated, the "source" domain and the "target" domain. The target domain is the problematic cognitive structure or process, which may have been identified by client and/or therapist. The source domain may originate from either client or therapist, and will typically have a concrete, experiential basis, and be easily pictured or simulated in imagery. In addition, it will often be shared between the client and the therapist (though this is not a prerequisite). Each of these domains may require elaboration, facilitated by the therapist. Then follows a process of cognitive synthesis, bridging the two domains and integrating meaning elements of each.

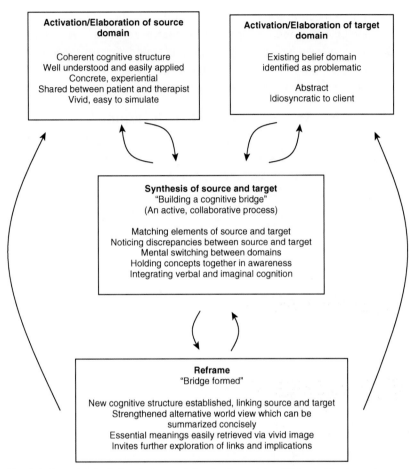

Fig. 2.1 A model depicting processes of activation, elaboration, synthesis, and reframe during metaphor use in therapy.

This process is likely to involve some sustained attention to both the verbal and imaginal components of each domain, switching between the two and allowing both to be entertained in conscious awareness. A new, cross-fertilized structure is thereby created, which may contain both verbal and imaginal components, and may stimulate further consideration and/or elaboration of each of the source and the target domains in a cyclical process. The degree to which these cognitive processes occur spontaneously, or require explicit therapist direction and facilitation, may vary enormously, and are part of the "art" of metaphor use, which will be elaborated in the next chapter. Finally, if successful, the client will leave with a reframed perspective on the problematic domain—a "strengthened alternative world view." This often invites further exploration of the links and implications of the metaphor, leading to further elaboration of source and/or target as well as further synthesis. In addition, a distinctive image will be captured in the client's mind, for ready future recall and allowing swift retrieval of the essential meanings involved. The metaphor provides a powerful therapeutic hook on which to hang future work.

Putting it together—an example of "grasping"

It might be useful to illustrate the workings of this model of metaphor use with one example. Imagine that a client, Matthew, says that he has a problem in "grasping ideas," which makes him feel inadequate in the workplace. The therapist asks him:

"What do you mean by grasping an idea? Is it like grasping an object?"

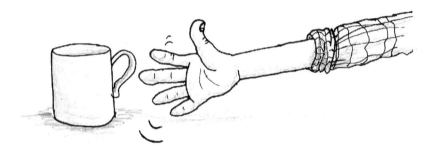

1. *Activation.* In asking Matthew this question, the therapist is activating the source domain of "object grasping." This cognitive structure contains well-developed sensorimotor imagery, grounded in experience, and is easy to simulate mentally. In addition, it is likely to be shared between Matthew and his therapist. Matthew needs to explore this imagery in order to understand what his therapist is asking. He imagines grasping a cup in his mind's eye. The therapist's question also ensures the target domain is activated, i.e. feeling inadequate in the workplace at not being able to grasp ideas.

2. *Elaboration.* The therapist's question makes Matthew enquire of himself what he does actually mean by difficulty grasping an idea. He elaborates the target domain in his mind, by trying to recall some recent times when he has sat in his office feeling miserable because he felt he was not on top of things.

3. *Synthesis.* Matthew tries to hold the two concepts in mind. While imagining grasping the cup, he also imagines trying to grasp an idea, and alternates between these simulations. As Matthew holds these images in mind, he matches elements between source and domain, and starts to see how the cup is an idea

at work and his hand is his mind trying to grapple with it. The metaphor begins to "fit" for him. However, the elements of the metaphor that do not fit—the error—now come to mind. Matthew gets the impression of being overwhelmed by ideas, but never is he overwhelmed by cups! What elaboration of the source domain would accommodate this? Perhaps the cups are now coming towards him on a conveyor belt and he doesn't have the time to grasp all of them. Matthew discusses this idea with his therapist in a cyclical process of elaboration and metaphoric synthesis. During this process, the client maintains the embodied simulation within their mind's eye, inspects it following questions from the therapist, and allows the image to change if this seems helpful. The therapist asks: "Do you have to grab all of these cups? What happens if you let some pass?" Matthew sees the cups huddling up in front of him, about to fall of the conveyor belt, which he tells the therapist. The therapist asks if there is an alternative option for the cups: "Is there somewhere else for them to go?" The client reports that actually some of the cups can go round the conveyor belt and back again—he hasn't missed them completely. The therapist asks: "Do you think ideas can be like this too?"

4. *Reframe.* Through elaboration and synthesis of these components, Matthew has developed a new cognitive structure functioning as a reframed perspective for his difficulties. There is a distinctive imaginal component, that of a circular conveyor belt of cups, some of which are selected, and others which go round. There are also some new thoughts. It is normal for there to be a plethora of ideas in the workplace. The most important can be acquired right away, and others will return at a later time, for future discussion. This provides Matthew with the impetus for a new set of cognitive and behavioural plans. He will remember this metaphor whenever he feels overwhelmed at work. He determines to select which concepts seem most important at the time and focus upon these. He no longer fears that ideas only come once, thereby getting bogged down in extraneous detail. He begins to notice that other colleagues don't get everything first time either, and that recaps, reminders, refreshers, and seeking advice are quite commonplace. Collaboratively, Matthew and his therapist have created a therapeutic hook, which they dub *conveyor belt ideas*, on which future work may be hung, both inside and outside the sessions.

It was suggested earlier that many of the source domains used in metaphor have a concrete, experiential basis. However, it should be noted that Matthew had most likely never been confronted with a conveyor belt of cups before! Indeed, many of the metaphors in this book use source domains that are not a familiar part of a person's every day experience, such as elephants, rockets, mythical characters, and so forth. Nevertheless, it is suggested that their important constituent components still retain a concrete and grounded experiential

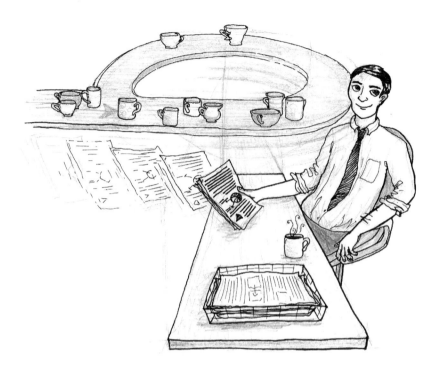

nature, often such as movement, direction, form, or growth. In Matthew's example, his familiarity with cups, grasping, objects in motion, and cyclical motion, made this metaphor feel grounded and easy to simulate mentally.

The process of inspection of a visual metaphor, allowing it to synthesize and transform within awareness is a process that needs to be understood from a conceptual angle—it seems to be at the heart of the therapeutic use of metaphors. It has a lot in common with imagery restructuring techniques. It seems to involve a broadening and sustaining of attention to percepts within imagination. It also seems to involve the client allowing change in imagery, some of which is guided, some of which may be random and nondirected. It would be beyond the remit of this book chapter to try and fully explain this process here. However, the interacting cognitive subsystems model may provide part of the framework—it proposes that the alternation between propositional (often verbal) and implicational (often embodied) meanings plays a core role in the transformation of meaning that aids recovery (Teasdale and Barnard, 1993). In terms of trying to conceptualize the mechanism of how perception can be controlled within imagination, a theory known as perceptual control theory (PCT; Powers, 1973, 2005) may be helpful. The relationship between this theory and psychological distress is described elsewhere (Mansell, 2005). For the purposes of this chapter, it is worth noting that it proposes that problems are solved through directing awareness towards the perceptual features of the problem, and that the resolution to the problem often emerges through "reorganization"—a randomly generated trial-and-error process.

Summary

This chapter has introduced the concept of metaphor use, and looked at its historical roots, theory, and conceptualization in cognitive therapy. A brief look at the history of metaphor showed how it has exercised minds as far back as Aristotle, and, in elemental form, may have origins way back in prelinguistic cognition. It has long been known how metaphor has great persuasive capacity, and unsurprisingly therapists of many orientations have wished to harness this power to therapeutic ends in their clients. More recent study has demonstrated the generative, constructive nature of metaphor, and how metaphor is inherent in much human discourse. Indeed, it is seen by many not only a natural, but also an essential vehicle through which to comprehend, think about and communicate the more abstract, and complex facets of ourselves and our world. Metaphor provides for us a cognitive bridge between our more concrete, familiar, experiential world, and the more abstract, opaque concepts and constructs with which we grapple.

There remains a great deal to be done in order to develop a fully integrated conceptual framework to understand metaphors. Nevertheless, we have proposed a working theoretical model comprising four essential processes in metaphor use, namely activation, elaboration, synthesis, and reframe. We are some way from a comprehensive understanding of all the component processes involved here, or indeed to answer important questions about which people may benefit more than others from a metaphorical approach in therapy. However, it is likely that certain key cognitive factors are involved: the willingness to try to understand a problem, the use of mental imagery, the integration between imagery, and verbal thought, the process of logging similarities between concepts despite superficial differences, the acceptance and use of multiple meanings, the broadening and sustaining of attention, and the facilitation of changes in perception within awareness. Now we have examined the theoretical basis for metaphor use, we must now turn attention to the different clinical ways in which it is skilfully employed. The "practice" of metaphor use is the subject of the next chapter.

Chapter 3

Clinical use of metaphor

Introduction

Chapter 2 provided a historical overview, leading to a theoretical account of the way metaphors can be applied in the context of cognitive therapy. It is clear that, throughout recorded history and almost certainly long before, metaphor has been actively used as a way of helping people to take a different perspective on the world and what it means. In particular, the use of metaphor can help people develop ways of thinking more clearly about how their world really works, as opposed to how they imagine or fear that it works. The constructive and therapeutic use of metaphor allows them to "step outside" their immediate preoccupations in ways which can increase their cognitive flexibility so that they can see things in a different and more helpful light than before, and, crucially, do so in ways that may enable them to try out different ways of responding to it in terms of meaning and behaviour. As a tool in cognitive therapy, direct or subtly used as described in this book, metaphor can make it possible for the person to free themselves from the chains imposed by counterproductive reactions and exercise choices that previously seemed impossible.

The applications of metaphor are diverse, and the specifics are rich and varied, as will be clear from the chapters which follow. The details of *how* metaphor can be used range from being highly prescriptive and directive through to highly interactive, exploratory, and subtle. Metaphors are invariably used in cognitive therapy as a way of interacting therapeutically in order to assist people to explore and come to understand existing unhelpful meanings and begin to think about things in a different way by constructing new, alternative meanings. In this chapter, the practicalities of applying this theoretical understanding will be outlined.

Principles of metaphor use in CBT: Why it can be helpful

Mechanism of change in the use of metaphor in CBT: Clinical applications

However metaphor is applied in practice, it will almost always involve a discussion in which the client is (implicitly or explicitly) helped to compare something that they *do not understand* (or understand in an incomplete, negative and/or unhelpful way) with something different *which they understand well.* This process makes it possible to offer a different, more helpful perspective than the person previously had. It is thus used to help the person to explore an entirely new or modified understanding of the problems they are experiencing in ways that may not only improve their understanding but also help them to choose to react differently. This is a key part of the bridge building function of therapeutic metaphor.

The use of metaphor can have the effect of allowing the person to try to make sense of what is happening to them and how they might deal better with their situation by invoking a comparison with something familiar that does not carry the same immediately distressing implications. That is, by considering and discussing a metaphor, the person is better able to process their interaction with the therapist regarding their problems and distress without their judgement being clouded or diverted by the unpleasant emotions they typically associate with the specific negative meanings involved in their distress. This does not, of course, mean that metaphors are free of emotions; metaphors often concern emotional situations and themes, and they may be vivid and emotionally charged. Sometimes it is helpful to deliberately choose emotional metaphors as a way of engaging the person more fully in the issues. Note that this may be negative or positive or even joyful; for example, comparing the anxiety and distress of confronting one's fears with giving birth; sometimes, it is necessary to struggle with discomfort and pain in order to fulfil our dreams.

Part of the basis for the use of metaphors in therapy is to allow the person to temporarily achieve some distance from their enmeshed and apparently uncontrollable emotional reactions with a view to being able to reengage with their problems from the different perspective offered by the metaphor discussed in therapy. This all contributes to helping the person to assimilate what they have learned in therapy into a new and more helpful view of the world and their place in it.

There is a further major advantage to using metaphor as part of CBT. Therapy is valuable not only in terms of the new understanding or "insight" that it helps bring to the client's view of their situation, but also in terms of enabling the client to apply and integrate these new perspectives into their daily life, their future therapy sessions, and to provide them with ways of explaining their new understanding to others. Crucial to this is the fact that the clinical use of metaphor usually serves to *enhance memory.* The person is better able to recall the vivid metaphor (precisely because it is so vivid), and at the same time to recall the well-integrated discussion surrounding the application of the metaphor to their situation and the new meanings that they acquired in the process. That is, the metaphor *primes* and *connects* the new meaning structure, which was identified as part of the discussion, making the parts more likely to elicit the whole, and allowing easy transitions between propositional and implicational levels of meaning (Teasdale, 1993).

The positive memory effects of metaphors can be further enhanced in a range of ways, including the use of different sensory and cognitive modalities, for example linking the metaphor to vivid visual imagery or existing strong memories or values, or to physical posture or actions. They can also be enhanced by mixing the familiar with the unusual and incongruous, attaching the metaphor to frequently occurring aspects of the person's daily life and behaviour and so on. Delivery of the metaphor through guided discovery, where the client actively participates in the exploration and negotiation of the metaphor and its application to their clinical problems, will enhance depth of processing, which in turn increases ease of retrieval, including the implicational meanings.

The style of delivery of the metaphor can also increase other aspects of memorability; for example, the therapist might enact some aspect of the scene (in the "broken leg" example below, the therapist might stand up and mimic walking with a plaster cast at an appropriate point in the discussion; in the "builder's apprentice" example on p. 137 as standing holding a wall will provide a vivid visual cue). Using a particular tone of voice (shouting or whispering) serves a similar function; for example, when an anxiety problem is personified as a metaphorical "bully" forcing the client to engage in safety seeking behaviour, (p. 145) an appropriately bullying tone of voice can be used to strengthen the conceptualization; the therapist indicates that the anxiety works by "ordering" the client to "obey" anxious commands (*Don't you dare stop worrying! It's only worrying a lot which keeps you safe! Isn't it?*).

Note that later in therapy, as the client tries to overcome their problems by changing what they do, the voice of the bully (and visual aspects of this metaphor as appropriate) can be deliberately visualized as becoming quieter, less certain, smaller, and otherwise less compelling. Sometimes this occurs spontaneously; a client with Obsessive Compulsive Disorder (OCD) who was confronting their obsessional fears as part of CBT said: "Every time I go against it, I think of the OCD shrinking into a corner and going "AAAAAaaaaaaargh". As he said this, the client mimes the shrinking OCD, holding out its hands protectively. He also says this with a sense of glee, his confrontation of his fears eliciting a sense of triumph linked to feelings of success and happiness. This example also illustrates the way in which metaphor can introduce elements of humour and fun into therapy (see later discussion).

Another strategy that can enhance processing, absorption of meaning and memory encoding is that of role-play, where the client is helped to actively participate in exploring the understanding offered by the metaphor by responding to or posing questions in the imaginary situation. In the "bully" example (p. 145), where we explore the way in which fear of negative consequences can motivate counterproductive behaviour, the therapist might adopt the role of the client's son (or some other child known to the client):

"Daddy, I need some money to give to a big boy at school to make sure that he doesn't hit me. Can I have some money please?"

(response from client...)

"Why not?"

(further discussion)

During the discussion and role-play, the therapist should make the link to the issues being referred to in the metaphor to ensure that the client is making the appropriate connections. In this case, the client is asked "how is OCD like a bully in your life?"

Exercises in which a systematic and explicit comparison between the problem and its metaphorical equivalent is made may also be helpful; for example, how does a bully work? How does OCD work? What happens if you give in to a bully? What happens if you give in to OCD? And so on. In this example, the therapist might do this as a written exercise on the whiteboard in their office or as homework on paper. "First write down how a bully tries to get what they want, then how it affects the person bullied. Next, write down how OCD tries to get what it wants, then how it affects the person with OCD......" and so on.

The use of vivid metaphors of this type is also helpful in reminding the client of what they have learned. By asking the client about the metaphor, they effectively prime the implicational meaning that the metaphor sought to convey. Thus, later in therapy, the client or therapist might say "that's just like when we talked about the bully." In this way, the vivid and unusual aspects of the metaphor aid in the retrieval of key meanings in therapy without the need for lengthy recapitulation.

The practicalities of metaphor use in CBT

The importance of the therapist–client interaction: negotiation and guided discovery

The use of metaphor in CBT requires a sometimes complex and always well-integrated *interaction* between client and therapist in order to understand better the way in which the client sees their situation and to help them to arrive at new, alternative, and most importantly, constructive ways of understanding and interacting with their world, internal and external. This can be viewed (metaphorically) as a negotiation, where therapist and client share their ideas about the metaphor and discuss, to and fro, how the metaphor might apply to the issues under consideration. As with any negotiation, it is helpful to sum-marize the agreed conclusion once negotiations are complete. The other com-monly used (often implicit) metaphor is the way in which therapy is conducted as guided discovery. Several aspects of identifying and clinically using metaphor described in this book are ways of conducting such guided discovery.

The fundamental principles of the use of metaphor in CBT, as outlined in the present chapter, are relatively straightforward. However, implementing them can be complex *for the therapist*, but should never be for the client. From the therapist's point of view, one can think of this process as being like a swan gliding upstream. It looks easy, graceful, and effortless. To make it happen, at least some of the time the swan is having to paddle furiously under the water! Making a metaphor work in a "natural" setting often requires considerable effort and thought on the part of the therapist. Metaphors are often multiuse; note that the swan metaphor, describing the process of therapy, can be clini-cally applied to a number of circumstances (e.g. in social phobia) where a client who managed a situation well initially discounts their success by com-paring how they felt with how other people appear ("No-one else looked as if they were trying as hard as I was"; "OK, but how much would others have seen that you were trying? Was it like the swan example we previously discussed? In what way?"). This example also illustrates that fact that metaphors can and should be adapted for different purposes as therapy progresses.

Using a metaphor to kick start therapy

To illustrate these points, an account of the use of a metaphor used as part of "guided discovery" illustrates the clinical use of a metaphor to aid understand-ing and engagement.

A client meets with a CBT therapist for the first session, and explains that they have actively chosen to come to CBT because, on the Internet, they found that CBT was the psychological therapy with the best evidence base for their problem. However, they had also read some critiques and were aware that cognitive therapists tended to focus on the "here and now," present-day man-ifestations and symptoms, and that this neglected the root causes of the prob-lem. So, can he please have CBT, but mainly focussing on the root causes rather than just symptoms?

Although this was not what the therapist has in mind for treatment, rather than arguing, the therapist responds through "guided discovery," drawing upon an explicit metaphor.

Therapist: Perhaps you are right. Let's think about this. I'd like you to imagine that you wake up tomorrow in hospital, and to your surprise, you are told your leg is broken. The emergency doctors ask you how your leg came to be broken. You can't recall, and you have a big bump on your head and a bit of a headache; it feels as if maybe your banged your head too, so can't recall the accident. When you tell your doctors, how will they react? Will they say "If we don't know what happened, we can't fix your leg'? Why not?

Client: [Explains that is not necessary for the cause to be known to deal with a broken leg.]

Therapist: CBT is a bit like that. However, did you know that doctors don't fix broken legs? In fact, broken legs heal. What doctors do is to see if there is anything which will interfere with your leg healing; for example, that the bones are not close to each other, or are at an angle. So, what they do is examine your leg in detail. They might even X-ray it, then do things to correct the problems that would stop your leg from healing, such as a plaster cast to keep the broken ends together so the bone can grow and join them. That's very similar to the kind of things we do in CBT.

Client: [interactive discussion with therapist]

Therapist: I want to work with you to find out whether there are things that might interfere with you being able to get over your problem and regain areas of your life you might have lost. Does that make sense?

Client: [more interactive discussion]

Therapist: Let's return to your original issue. You mentioned the importance of understanding causes, and I think it sometimes might be important. Think about the broken leg situation. When its time to leave the hospital to go back to your home (where it seems likely your leg got broken in the first place), I'm wondering if there might be good reasons to consider what happened to break it?

Client: [concludes, sometimes with gentle prompting, that the reasons would be "to make sure it doesn't happen again"].

Therapist: Yes. Perhaps it was just bad luck, you tripped over your own foot. But....perhaps there is a loose piece of stair carpet; if you don't spot it and nail it down, then you might find that you have a similar accident in the future. Something similar applies to CBT; as we go through therapy aimed at helping you deal with your problems on a day to day basis, we will be on the lookout for things which might have been involved in why you developed the problem. Perhaps it was just bad luck, or perhaps we can identify particular issues which need to be dealt with.

Note that later in treatment the therapist might wish to discuss themes and assumptions that have repeatedly emerged in the course of sessions, so he or she would say "Do you recall that at the beginning of treatment we talked about the importance of things that might have been involved in triggering your problem by comparing it to the situation where you had a broken leg?" followed by the idea of needing to deal with the loose piece of stair carpet in order to prevent problems recurring in the future.

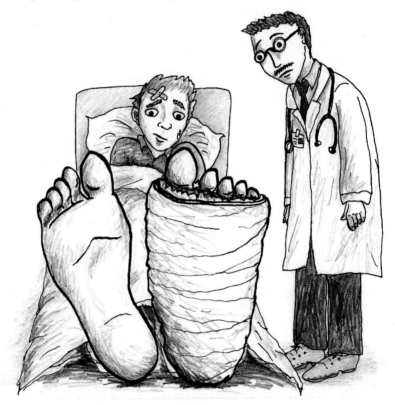

This example illustrates some of the key issues in the clinical use of metaphors in CBT as already described above. As described above, the essence of the therapeutic use of metaphor and analogies is that the person's problem, or some aspect of it, is compared to something quite different and easier to understand. This is done in order to stimulate discussion and, as part of that discussion, build the "cognitive bridge," which increases the person's understanding of their problem, how it works, and how it might be dealt with.

One might reasonably ask: how does this clarify rather than confuse? Surely it would be better to talk about the problem itself as in "psychoeducation," directly describing the workings of the brain and mind, without using comparisons with things not directly relevant to the person's distress, suffering, and psychological pain?

Distress, suffering, and psychological pain can have the effect of making it harder for the affected person to think clearly about what is happening to them, whereas in some instances, the use of a metaphor is less emotionally laden and helps the person to take a different perspective. The use of metaphor in the context of "guided discovery" is in turn linked to the key goal of reaching a "shared understanding" of the client's problems; the way a metaphor stimulates discussion leads the client to recognize the formulation as being something that they worked with the therapist to generate (see p. 38 below).

The shared understanding can then be explored and applied by the client with help from their therapist; the main application is to place the person in the position of being able to choose to change how they react, and to give them a framework to evaluate the effects and results of the changes they seek to make. The therapist helps them to consider that it might be possible to think about their situation differently and possibly more helpfully, adopting the more active position of experimenting with, seeking to control and acting on their situation rather than simply reacting to it. They become an explorer or scientist, findings out new things about their world and their place in it.

This guided discovery based approach, with appropriate use of metaphors, contrasts sharply with the simplistic notion that CBT involves telling the client that their thinking is incorrect, illogical, irrational, or otherwise "wrong" and teaching them better thinking skills so as to encourage more positive thinking and so on. The person is encouraged and helped to view their problem *from a different perspective*, or even a range of different perspectives. As described in Chapter 2, several metaphors might be used in parallel in order to illustrate and explore different aspects of the problem that the therapist and client are working together to try to understand and change.

The importance of identifying and balancing emotions

Although metaphors can be helpful in allowing clients to engage in consideration of issues that would otherwise be emotionally overwhelming, it is important to emphasize that accessing emotional material is a key part of the way in which cognitive therapy is done. Metaphors can be used to strike the right balance between keeping the discussion emotionally engaged and making sure that things do not "boil over."

Most therapists will be familiar with the phenomenon of the client who tries to "rationalize" their problem, and in doing so actually avoids thinking too deeply or closely about their problems. For example, an anxious client who experiences panic attacks says "I know that nothing bad will happen. My doctor has told me that I'm not going to faint or go mad, and I'm sure that's right. However, it's hard to convince myself of that when it happens."

In this case, the client is encouraged to explore their fears by the therapist saying

"I know that that's what is in your head, what you tell yourself even when you are panicking. What's in your head is very important, but I'm wondering, when you think back to your last panic attack, what did you really believe, *in your heart*, was the worst thing that could happen right then at that moment?"

Locating feelings and ideas in different places to the one the client uses to cope can be helpful in a range of ways. The obsessional client, who makes it clear that they believe that their ideas of harming their loved ones is senseless, is asked "when you are filled with fear, what kind of ideas lurk in the back of your mind?" Other examples are "What is your gut feeling?" and "What's going on in the dark recesses of your mind?"

Some clients use a stream of self-reassuring thoughts to try to combat the fears which they try to prevent taking them over as they see it. This leads to experiential avoidance, which serves to maintain or even increase the person's distress, while they remain convinced that the opposite is true. It is helpful both to identify the phenomenon and to show how the counterproductive elements work. For example, a depressed client, in their thought recording, indicates that, when they were particularly depressed a few days before their main thoughts were:

"Don't worry."
"It will all turn out fine."
"I've done my very best."
"No, I am definitely not a failure."
"I will cope."
"Things are not as bad as they seem."

At first glance, these seem helpful thoughts of the kind that a therapist might help the client to use to help them feel better. However, more careful consideration reveals these to be self-reassurance thoughts, where the patients try to "argue themselves better" by simply contradicting their negative thinking. Asking for belief ratings might help identify this. Another way of helping the client to make sense of what is happening is to compare this recorded sequence to an *overheard phone conversation*.

"It's like I just came into the room and you were talking on the telephone. Those thoughts you wrote down: those are your 'end of the conversation'. It seems like you're having a bit of an argument down the phone. What I'd like to know is what the other end of the argument is. These things that you're saying seem to be answers to some other ideas which you have in your head. Think back to the time you wrote these things; what was going through your mind that you felt you had to answer in this way?"

The therapist may sometimes describe the process of change and what is needed to take place as being like taking things from "head to heart," sometimes with a gesture, the therapist touching their forehead then moving their hand to the left-hand side of their chest.

Metaphor and understanding the cognitive theory of emotions and emotional disorders

The use of metaphor in CBT is embedded in the fundamentals of cognitive theory. The essential idea underpinning Beck's (1976) cognitive model of emotion is that a person's emotional reactions are a function of the way in which they organize reality and attribute meaning to events and situations; that is, how they make sense of their world and therefore how they interpret or appraise their moment-by-moment experience. It is, of course, the *meaning* of what happens that elicits emotions rather than events themselves. For example, a photograph of a person's happy wedding day may move them to sad tears after the death of the loved one. The particular appraisal made in any given situation thus depends on the context in which an event occurs, the person's preexisting emotional state at the time, and their values, past experiences, and beliefs. The cognitive theory specifies that specific emotions "belong" to particular types of interpretations. Effectively this means that the same event can evoke a different emotion in different people, or even different emotions in the same person on different occasions. This *abstract idea* of cognition-emotion specificity can be illustrated by a more *concrete story* (adapted from Salkovskis, 1996); it concerns dog mess.

Therapist: As I left for work this morning, three other men were setting out at the same time. By coincidence, the same thing happened to each of us. As each walked out of his house, we all stood in some dog mess. For the first person, his past experience meant that the he has a bit of a tendency to feel depressed. His immediate reaction when he looked down at his shoes was typical of how he tended to think; he thought: "I am a failure. I used to be successful, but now something as simple as leaving my own house becomes a disaster. There is no point in my continuing; this is just typical of what the rest of the day is going to be like." Feeling very depressed, this person went back to bed.

The second person had the same unpleasant experience, but reacted quite differently. Being prone to anxiety, this person's reaction was: "What am I going to do? If I go back in the house and wash this off I will be late for my meeting with my boss, and so I'll lose my job. On the other hand, if I don't, then I'll stink, and the boss will decide that I have a personal hygiene problem and I will lose my job anyway".

We leave this person in a state of indecision and find that the third person has also encountered the dog mess. Now this person tends to have a problem with anger, and this occasion is no exception. Their immediate (loud!) thought is, "*Whose dog did this??? How many times must I tell my neighbors not to allow their dog to stop outside my house but, oh no, do they listen? You wait 'til I catch who's responsible for this, they're in for real trouble!*"

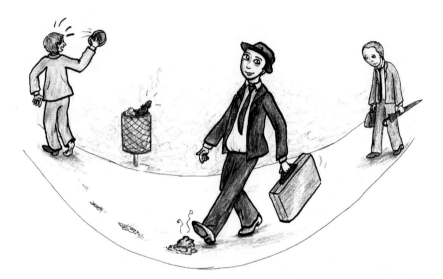

This story neatly illustrates Beck's principle of specificity, with feelings of depression associated with ideas of loss, feelings of anxiety associated with ideas of personal danger or threat, and anger with ideas that someone else has been unfair or broken one's personal rules. Guilt involves the belief that we have broken our own rules. (see also Beck's burglar example, Chapter 4, p. 58).

This story can be used in therapy to illustrate emotional responding. Having considered (and in therapy, discussed) the implications of this story for the way emotion is understood, the metaphor can, if useful, be further developed to illustrate and unfold a further point, this time about the underpinnings and philosophy of therapy. The story continues on the basis that the author, a cognitive therapist, is not immune to standing in dog mess, and so on.

Therapist: As I left the house myself (and let's be clear that I'm perfectly capable of stepping in dog mess from time to time) the same thing happens to me. However, my reaction is yet again different. Looking down at my feet, I smile and think "Thank goodness I didn't put on sandals this morning."

The implications of this second part of the metaphor can now be drawn out. This aspect of the story suggests several things; firstly, that cognitive therapy is not necessarily about thinking more rationally or more positively (although both might happen as a result of CBT). Secondly, it clearly suggests instead the idea that there may be several *alternative* ways of looking at any particular situation or problem. It is explained that cognitive therapists take the view that people who experience emotional difficulties are often (and perhaps always) stuck in a particularly negative or unhelpful way of looking at their situation, and they implicitly regard their reactions as the "true" or only way of interpreting what is happening. Note that, when helping the client to consider the need for alternative accounts, metaphors of being "stuck" can be very helpful in making sense of their present position.

In such circumstances, being told that one's thinking is irrational or illogical is implicitly critical, and is dangerously close to being simply told to "pull yourself together." The person may become more unhappy and feel more trapped, because they can see that there is a problem, that it might involve them being illogical or perhaps even stupid, but without being able to either understand it or begin to see a solution. They may even conclude that there might not be a solution. "Doctor, even my own thinking is against me … this is terrible. What can I do?"

How therapy works: Formulation, the alternative explanation and beyond

The metaphor used above should make it clear that the role of the cognitive therapist is to help the person explore whether or not there might be alternative ways of appraising and understanding the situation they find themselves in; this is what the cognitive formulation or "shared understanding" is for. The person is helped to identify where (and how) they may have become "trapped" or "stuck" in their way of thinking, and then to allow them to identify and consider other ways of looking at their situation, particularly examining more helpful ways of reacting both in general and to specific situations or experiences.

Good therapy thus involves helping the client to make sense of *how the world really works*; this means both the person's internal and external worlds, and represents a substantial change from the inflexible set of negative beliefs that characterize emotional disorders. The identification, generation, and exploration of metaphors can be particularly helpful in this shift, because when used properly metaphors allow the client and therapist to identify, discuss and make sense of other perspectives about what is happening which make sense to both (Salkovskis, 1996). Metaphors allow them to construct a flexible model with implications both for understanding and change.

Another metaphor is helpful here. The partner and best friend metaphor helps understanding of the relevance of having an "alternative explanation" as opposed to being reassured; that is, being told that one's negative beliefs are incorrect. The person is asked to imagine that they are sitting at home when their partner's mobile telephone receives a text.

"You notice that the text on your partner's phone is from your best friend, and says 'can you meet me at 4 pm rather than 5 pm tomorrow?'. This is a surprise, as you don't know about any meeting. Even more surprisingly, you notice that there are several other texts, also referring to meetings over the last few weeks that you were not aware of; some of them say 'are you sure that they don't know?' and 'will they be away then?', obviously referring to yourself. There are also several phone calls. If this was you, what would you be worried about?"

Usually, the worry is that they are having an affair. The metaphor proceeds:

"So you mention what you noticed on their phone to your partner, and they seem a bit irritated. They categorically tell you not to be silly; there is nothing going on. They are vehement about this, and indicate that they are upset that you think otherwise."

The person has now been "reassured" by her partner; surely this is enough? If not, why not?

Bear in mind that such reassurance is commonly the main help that is offered to people with psychological problems. People are told that they are not a failure and that the danger they fear will not happen and so on. As we know, in severe and persistent problems, such reassurance is not only ineffective, but can make things worse. For example, repeated reassurance in health anxiety and OCD can be compared to "digging to get out of a hole" (see Chapter 7, p. 145).

Why is reassurance not enough in that instance? The point here is, of course, that being told that "there is nothing to worry about" is bland and empty, because it provides no explanation of what is happening and why. That is, it does not offer a convincing alternative account of *what is really going on.* Reassurance (that your fears are groundless, for example) can sometimes can help one feel a bit better, but what is really needed is something that allows the person to take a different and less negative view of the source of their concerns. In the example here, it continues:

"Two weeks after this incident (and the unhelpful reassurance) you come home one night to find the house crowded with your friends. It's your birthday, and your partner and your best friend have been secretly arranging a surprise party for you. Now you know this, your anxiety and suspicions disappear; it all makes sense."

The partner and best friend metaphor suggests that what is needed is a clear and understandable alternative explanation to allow the person to "let go" of the unhelpful negative beliefs. What is the alternative explanation in cognitive therapy? The answer, of course, is the formulation.

Persons and Tompkins (2007) described formulation as a key element of empirical hypothesis testing, which is comprised of assessment leading to formulation that suggests interventions, which in turn feeds back into the formulation. Bieling and Kuyken (2003, p.53) suggest that "Cognitive case formulation can be defined as a coherent set of explanatory inferences about the factors causing and maintaining a person's presenting problems, inferences derived from the cognitive theory of emotional disorders."

Butler (1998) describes formulation as a metaphorical map that is a way of viewing a client's difficulties. The metaphorical idea of a map, which places the client and therapist in the role of explorers with different areas of expertise, which will help in their explorations, is particularly helpful as a way of thinking about formulation. It suggests that the map (formulation) may initially be sketchy, incomplete, and wrong in places. Nevertheless it can provide the basis for exploration and discovery, which will lead to corrections in the map and more confident further exploration. The map is a way of recording what is already known and finding new directions to travel. The formulation is thus seen as both collaborative and evolving, and provides a guide as to how treatment might progress (see also Chapter 4, p. 56).

Thus, during the assessment and formulation (developing shared understanding) stages of therapy, as part of the process of guided discovery, the therapist works with the client to weave together two sets of information: on the one hand, the therapist's understanding of the client's problems within the context of the cognitive model of emotional problems and on the other the client's experience of these problems. The result is a picture of how the problem might work. The therapist then helps the person identify any obstacles there might be to thinking and acting in the more helpful ways that the client might wish to choose, and to examine ways of overcoming such obstacles. Thus, cognitive therapy is a fundamentally empowering approach that aims to help the client to free themselves to identify and validate other ways of interpreting their situation and reacting to it, drawing from the fullest possible range of alternatives available to them (including their current negative account).

Therapy seeks to broaden the choices the person can make about the way they react to their situation, and helping them to discover information which allows them to decide between the available choices in an informed way. It may well be that the chosen alternative is more rational, it might even be more positive, but it does not have to be. This philosophy highlights the importance of *guided discovery* where the therapist helps the person themselves to explore alternative ways of looking at their situation. By definition, this style of therapy also means that the alternatives arrived at are acceptable to the client and consistent with their beliefs and values. Metaphor can be used as a tool both to increase understanding and explore the implications the new understanding offered through guided discovery.

Selecting the right metaphor

An important task for the therapist is to select a metaphor or metaphors that are meaningful to the client, as the example chosen must resonate sufficiently to ensure processing and understanding. Not uncommonly, clients will substitute the therapist's example with a more salient one of their own—this is great and should be encouraged (see also the discussion of client-generated metaphors, p. 45). It is helpful to make sure that the correct process or target has been identified; even if has not been, it can be useful to add the client's alternative metaphor to the current version of the shared understanding which has evolved in the course of therapy.

The second task is to help crystallize the core elements of a metaphor and link them to the specific issues for that client. Thirdly, once the client has understood the meaning of the metaphor in the particular context of how their problems works and/or how such problems might be tackled, it is important to help them test out both the validity and the implications of these conclusions. This might involve drawing on past their understanding of their past experience and wherever possible using behavioural experiments ("to find out how the world really works"). This process also assists in the transition "from head to heart." Note that sometimes these behavioural experiments can be "thought experiments"; e.g. the example (p. 44) in which it is suggested to an obsessional client (who fears that she is contaminated) that she might be useful to the government as an assassin; all she would need to do is to touch something, which will be later touched by the victim. To be most clinically useful, a metaphor usually needs to meet certain characteristics.

It must be readily understandable (or best of all, already understood) by the person to whom it is being offered. This means that the choice of metaphor should draw on the person's background and interests. Sometimes it is obvious, as the person themselves provides the metaphor or analogy, either implicitly through the use of a particular phrase ("I don't want to rock the boat"; see p. 147) or by directly describing one ("That makes me think of...." or

"It's just like......"). Knowledge of the person's background and interests are also helpful; people interested in computers or gardening will probably be helped by somewhat different analogies and metaphors. Some experiences are relatively universal and well understood by most (e.g. relationships, how children react).

"Dead metaphors," where the person uses a particular phrase that has become linguistically attached to a particular meaning although separated from the full metaphor, can also be helpful, especially if illustrated and grasped. (To "grasp" an idea is a good example of a dead metaphor, see p. 16). For example, people who fear that they will "go mad" or "have a nervous break-down" describe their concerns as "their mind will snap." The therapist discusses what they mean, and illustrates it by taking a pencil and breaking it in the session. It is suggested that, by using this implicit metaphor, the client has also adapted a (possibly mistaken) implication, which is that their mind will be broken beyond repair, like the two ends of the pencil the therapist is holding. They are invited to consider that perhaps the mind does not work that way. Feeling that one has "lost control" or that one has been "overwhelmed" may be more like bursting into tears; once the moment passes, you return to normal and may even feel better. Bursting into tears can be a sign of feeling over-whelmed, but is not in any way irreversible. Note also that the unusual action of deliberately breaking a pencil in two makes the metaphor more vivid and memorable.

Cross-cultural issues

Another important criterion with respect to the choice of metaphor is that its focus is consistent with the person's culture and value system. For example, normalizing reactions to stress can involve invoking the idea of an "evolution-ary heritage"; in the context of therapy, evolution is both a scientific founda-tion of human psychology and can be used as a highly effective metaphor. When one of the authors was discussing with a client the fact that feared situ-ations do not usually result in fainting, he said that this would not make sense for our ancestors; when confronted by a predator or enemy, fainting would be fatal. The client looked concerned, saying "as a Jehovah's Witness I don't accept evolutionary ideas," so the therapist simply switched to whether God would have made us to react in this way.

By definition, metaphors are embedded in the client's understanding of the world, which draws upon their background, including culturally specific understanding. As described in Chapter 2, a metaphor is likely to be more valuable and effective if its "source" material is well-understood and can be simulated readily by the listener. Note, however, that there is *not* a requirement that the individual has personally experienced the exact details of what is being described in the metaphor. For example, "elephants on train tracks" (see p. 138) is a powerful and accessible metaphor but is outside the experience of the vast majority of people from any culture. Similarly one may easily relate to the metaphor of a boat on a rough sea (p. 166) without having ever having been a seafarer. Indeed, many of the concrete "source materials" used in metaphor, including animals, plants, buildings, prisons, journeys, and the nature of up and down, transcend most cultural boundaries, though of course the individual details may vary widely. Similarly, many of the abstract concepts which form the "target" of much metaphor, such as causation, responsibility, or ambivalence, are also widely relevant to human beings whatever their cultural background, although again the details may vary widely.

One metaphor that helps counter any presumption that cultural differences represent a fundamental block to understanding is the "foreign market" metaphor. Compare the experience of going to a market in your home town and going to a market somewhere unfamiliar, say in China. When you go to the Chinese market, everything looks unfamiliar, even the writing. It is hard to see what this has in common with the market you know in Basingstoke, UK. However, if you look at it more closely, people are buying and selling things that are needed for everyday life. The seller makes a living by selling their wares, the buyer takes it home to cook for their family, and life goes more smoothly for all as a result. The *fundamentals* of the market are almost identical, but the *details* are very different. The same is true of psychological problems; the fundamentals are the same in social phobia in the United Kingdom, Botswana, and Japan, but the *details* are different, reflecting different social values. Could your client help you find your way round the foreign market? What might they need to explain to you so that you can make sense of it? Could they do the same thing in terms of your understanding of their problems?

Cognitive behavioural therapy, and particularly the collaborative, explicit approach to metaphor advocated in this book, lends itself well to the successful application of metaphor in a cultural context. A particular kind of relationship between therapist and patient is fostered which permits two-way dialogue and discussion. A metaphor can thus be "opened up" for discussion, "thrown onto the table" so to speak. Gentle enquiry can be made as to whether the metaphor "resonates" and whether the client relates to it. Sometimes the client may choose to substitute a variation of the metaphor, which more closely resembles an experience from their cultural repertoire, and this can be welcomed by the therapist. Crucially, the therapist does not take an "expert" stance but can show humility and curiosity—being genuinely interested in learning from the client's own superior knowledge of themselves and their culture, and then facilitating an adaptation of the metaphor to help achieve the fundamental shifts in meaning that are judged to be important.

Humour in metaphor and "spoiling the joke"

Sometimes metaphors take the form of jokes and humourous stories, as in the "dog mess" story earlier. Humour in therapy has to be used carefully, with the therapist's main concern being that the client may consider that the therapist is mocking or making fun of them, or being patronizing. Two factors are key: the context in which humour/jokes are used and the therapeutic relationship. The easiest case is "accidental" humour, where the client is amused by something they or the therapist said, making it easy for the therapist to join in. Typically, it is helpful in such circumstances, once the amusing moment has passed, to ask the question "Why is that funny?" Although it often spoils the joke (!), what it also does is help the client and therapist reflect on the perspective that has been gained to make something humourous. This is also true when humourous remarks or stories are more deliberately used. For example, an obsessional client feared that she might harm those she loved if she did not wash her hands in a prolonged and careful way, avoid touching potential contaminants, and so on. As part of the process of helping the client to engage in a behavioural experiment involving exposure and response prevention (touching a sandwich then eating it), the therapist said:

Therapist: Susan, I think you should consider a career change. You work on a supermarket checkout at the moment, and it's not particularly well paid. What I suggest is that we contact the secret service and offer your services as a special agent. Your job would be to go to diplomatic parties, then offer food to the "target" without first washing your hands. You could be an assassin!

Client: [laughs].

Therapist: Why is that funny?

Client: It's funny because you can't kill people like that.

In this example, the explicit dissection of the humour leads to a conclusion on the part of the client, which is ironic, given the precise focus of her OCD … that you *can* kill people like that! The discussion which followed culminated in the client touching snacks, eating some herself, and handing others out to the therapist and people in the clinic, and then repeating a similar exercise at home. This metaphor embodies the important issue that distressed clients often feel that they are responsible or to blame for things that they cannot or could not have control over, and the judicious use of humour has helped crystallize the key message.

Client-generated metaphors

Several characteristics of good metaphor have already been described, as well as the typically Socratic, collaborative approach to their exploration and application, the need for resonant and culturally meaningful metaphor, and the judicious use of humour. The building of "cognitive bridges," while always a joint undertaking, is often initiated by the therapist. However, many clients can and will spontaneously introduce their own metaphor into the therapeutic dialogue, often with similar intentions and motivations. They are trying to make sense of their difficulties, and quite naturally rely on metaphor to comprehend and communicate their predicament to the therapist. An important question therefore concerns how the therapist should handle any such *client-generated* metaphor; is their proposed cognitive bridge well-conceived, well-constructed, and helpful?

There are certainly good reasons to pay close attention to client-generated metaphor. First, such metaphor clearly already has the client's attention and often represents the client's attempts to make sense of an abstract problem. Second, the metaphor may reveal important meanings that were not previously apparent. Third, the imagery associated with the client's metaphor may be vivid and memorable, and thus continue to draw the client into thinking about their problem along these lines.

For example, take the metaphor offered by the woman mentioned in Chapter 2 (p. 6). For her, living life had always been like running as fast as possible up an escalator—unfortunately, however, it was a "down" escalator. This had been provided by the client in the context of an assessment—an attempt to capture and convey to her new therapist the essence of her plight over many years. It was clear this was not a passing flight of fancy; it had occurred to her before many times, and represented an enduring and persistent view of her struggles. This metaphor was vivid, and had her attention, so some time was spent unpacking its meanings. For her, many elements of life were nonsensical, contrary, and even "cruel." This included a critical work environment, and the seeming impossibility of achieving many of her cherished aspirations, such as meeting a partner or owning a place of her own. Why was she running up the escalator? Because she was trying hard, she was sticking to her guns, and was determined not to give up. And yet, her continued labour only resulted in more frustration and failure, reinforcing her view that the world was unfairly skewed against her. *It is not me that is going the wrong way,* she observed, *it is the escalator!*

One of the first challenges for the therapist, when confronted with a client-generated metaphor such as this, is to make a choice: Should the metaphor be extended, perhaps shaping it to convey more benign, helpful meanings, or should it be changed entirely? In bridge terminology, this is the choice of whether to help build, strengthen, and repair the cognitive bridge, keeping much of its essence, or to demolish and begin afresh. This can be a difficult decision. Sometimes the metaphor can appear destructive and entrenched, merely crystallizing a maladaptive view of the client or their world. However, for the reasons given earlier, there is often much attention, meaning, and imagery invested in the metaphor, and it may be discarded at considerable cost.

In the case of the woman and the escalator, the decision was made to extend and modify the metaphor, rather than abandon it. Several strands of therapeutic work contributed to a rationale for "restructuring" the metaphor, which was undertaken and refined in stages. In short, the client realized she was far from alone in finding many of life's challenges difficult. Also, she had some degree of agency in being able to choose environments which suited her. Also, there were many exceptions to the rule that "the world was against her." Such revisions of meaning translated into rather a different picture of the client and the escalator. Indeed, there were many more people in the scene, following different paths, with different wishes, and many escalators with different types, speeds, directions, and gradients. She realized it was her responsibility to find her own escalator, not to stay on one that didn't suit her.

The metaphoric transformation was only possible here once the meanings had been explored and restructured. Without this, the revised metaphor would be vacuous and unconvincing. The imagery transformation helped crystallize the metaphorical shift and had the added benefit that it could be rehearsed and embedded with relative ease. The client's emotional troubles were not over, at the point of embracing this new metaphor. However, the sense of passivity, frustration, and hopelessness had been removed sufficiently to motivate further cognitive and behavioural exploration of a new approach to viewing her world. She was able to be more assertive in seeking help, in making decisions and choices, in interacting with like-minded people, in dismissing frustrations, and not taking things personally.

Sometimes, however, the therapist needs to encourage a qualitative shift to a metaphor, which is more useful. One example concerns a client who declared that he was "a bomb waiting to go off." This particular client was concerned about his temper and irritability, and was keeping himself isolated from others because of a fear of "explosion." The catastrophic, irreversible, all-or-nothing nature of this metaphor was accompanied by a sense of utter passivity—the "waiting." The client was viewing himself as a dangerous entity, unsafe for human contact, and with no agency to alter the inevitable course of events. His therapist made a choice that the "bomb" metaphor had little long-term value and was potentially harmful, so explored with the client a possible alternative.

Client: I feel as if I am a bomb waiting to go off.

Therapist: You mean with your anger? That sounds pretty dramatic.

Client: Yes, I'm really scared—I'm not myself, I feel all pent up with anger with so many things—and no one else needs that. So I don't risk being around others.

Therapist: So it feels like you are a danger to be around other people?

Client: I guess. I would never want to hurt anyone, but I'm scared that one day I might just explode.

Therapist: In the past, what has happened when you've got angry?

Client: I feel worse and worse inside, like the blood is all rushing around in my head, and that makes me think more and more about it all.

Therapist: So actually you get into a vicious circle where you are feeling worse and worse, then spending more time dwelling on it in your head?

Client: Definitely.

Therapist: And then what happens?

Client: I dunno. Maybe something stops me, or I just shout "Stop it!" to myself.

Therapist: And then how do you feel?

Client: A little calmer. And then I usually try and do something different, distract myself.

Therapist: That's interesting. I can see that there's a lot "simmering away" inside you, but when it gets bad it sounds more like a pan of water which kind of "boils over" briefly, before simmering again?

Client: That's exactly right. I hate that.

Therapist: Sure, that must be really unpleasant for you. But I wonder if that "pan boiling over" idea fits with what's going on for you better than the "bomb going off" idea?

Client: Well, yes, maybe the bomb would never go off…

Therapist: Or maybe there is no bomb?

Client: Just a pan of water, you mean? Yes I see what you mean. Well I've never been violent. I just get these angry moments over and over again. How can I stop it?

Therapist: Well, supposing we go with the pan idea, for a minute. You said when you start to feel angry, you think more and more about it all.

Client: Yes, it just spirals.

Therapist: Right. So that's a bit like the pan of water getting hotter, and then you are turning up the heat even more?

Client: OK… so I need to turn the heat off?

Therapist: Well, absolutely, we might need to work together to find ways for you to lower the temperature when needed; so you are more in control of what is happening and not get overtaken by your anger.

Once again, this therapeutic exchange could not be expected to eliminate the client's anger or even maybe his anxiety about his anger. However, the therapist's decision to encourage a qualitative shift from a catastrophic, unhelpful metaphor about bombs to a more adaptive one about simmering pans and temperatures paves the way for a more hopeful, active, and promising piece of therapeutic work.

The meta-metaphor: CBT is a skilful blend of clinical art and clinical science

At its most fundamental, cognitive behavioural therapy involves a complex synthesis of several factors in ways which have the effect of helping people to deal more effectively with their psychological problems. These factors include the scientific understanding of factors involved in the way particular types of problems develop and are maintained across and within disorders, general principles of how meaning and behaviour can be changed, and the way such general factors result in highly specific manifestations in any particular person experiencing psychological distress. Add to this already complex mix the requirement for the therapist to possess good interpersonal understanding and be able to express this understanding in ways that help the client feel understood and empowered, to deploy these skills in ways which build a collaborative relationship, and to introduce specific strategies such as the use of metaphor to maximize the client's ability to benefit. This blend of clinical art and clinical science requires knowledge, skill, sensitivity, intuition, cognitive flexibility, and the ability of the therapist to put this all together. All of this is the context in which we have to place the use of metaphor in CBT; in this context metaphor cuts to the heart of the problem, while without it we have at best a blunt instrument.

Chapter 4

Principles, format, and context of CBT

Introduction

We covered the general principles of using metaphors in clinical practice in the last chapter. In this chapter we focus in further detail on how metaphors can be used to acquaint the client with the key elements of CBT itself. It is not always easy for a therapist to explain CBT to a client. The same problem occurs when trying to explain any complex system of principles and practice to someone who encounters it for the first time. Could you fully envisage a foreign country and its culture before travelling to that country and living there for a while? Can you imagine what it would like to work in another field—an air traffic controller, a barrister, or an actuary? Our clients may be faced with a similar, inevitable, lack of knowledge. At the best, they might have studied social science, or seen CBT practiced in an edited format on the television. At the worst, their image of a CBT therapist may be very similar to that of a stereotype of a Freudian analyst or even a medical doctor who "prescribes" psychological advice.

There is a good argument for allowing our clients to just "experience" CBT to work out what it is. However well you described the experiences during the first day at school, a wedding ceremony, or a bungee jump, this would never be a substitute for the real thing. Right? This analogy cuts both ways. Even though we do not expect a person to completely understand a wedding ceremony simply through being told about it—this is still a good start—and in real life people rarely face a situation without getting information first such as reading about it, or witnessing it happening to someone else. In this way, information may help a person to make an informed decision about whether to try the therapy, and prepare them for it. Clients will ask questions, and it is appropriate to try to answer them if it aids their understanding. A further reason for having ways of explaining CBT concepts is that it helps to frame what the therapist is actually doing within the therapy at that time. Thus, a questioning procedure, or a behavioural experiment, can be conducted with the client's full knowledge and consent as to its purpose.

This chapter focuses on the principles, format, and context of CBT, rather than on the psychological processes and theory that are thought to underlie its use. If CBT were football, the principles would refer to the rules of the game, e.g. to score as many goals as possible, the format would refer to the more concrete details, such as the number of players on each team, and the context would be its roles, i.e. as a participating sport, a visual spectacle, or as a career path. So how can we use metaphor to explain the first of these—the principles of CBT?

Principles of CBT

The therapeutic relationship

Arguably, the fundamental principle of CBT is the collaborative relationship between the therapist and the client. Any attempts at shifting patterns of thinking or behaviour ideally occur as part of an open, collaborative agreement, rather than something the therapist "does" to the client. This kind of relationship is often not expected by clients on commencing CBT, maybe because of their experience of controlling or manipulative relationships, or the cultural assumption of a therapist as a paternalistic figure who administers esoteric techniques such as hypnotism and free association. Therefore, it can help to have some analogies at hand to try to explain your role as a CBT therapist when these assumptions come into play, and interfere with the process of CBT. Clients may ask to be told what to do, or conversely, react negatively to what they perceive you are instructing them to do. In these situations, it can be difficult for the therapist to maintain a collaborative stance themselves, and find that they get drawn into providing advice or defending themselves. Therefore, it may be helpful for therapists themselves to have a metaphorical image of their role that they can use to anchor the relationship at these times. There are several metaphors we have encountered that illustrate different features of the therapeutic relationship.

Two experts

A good way of characterizing this special collaborative relationship is refer to therapy involving "two experts in the room." It is suggested that the therapist is an expert in emotional disorders, how they work, and how they might be treated. The therapist has little knowledge about the client and their life, and will need the client's help to understand this better. By contrast, the client is not only an expert on their life, but also in *their particular type of problem and how it works in the context of their life*. The client, of course, does not have as much expertise as the therapist in the understanding and treatment of the type of emotional problem they are experiencing and may need the therapist's help in understanding it better. In therapy therefore the aim is to bring together the two types of expertise.

Sometimes it may be valuable to elaborate the "experts" analogy further. The "architect and surveyor" metaphor helps achieve this vividly, again helping to challenge preconceptions that the therapist provides wisdom, magic, or paternalistic advice. An architect has the idea for a new, ecofriendly, exclusive house in a scenic meadow with beautiful meandering streams. He cannot build the house straight away. What would happen if the streams flooded, or if the house were to obstruct a major footpath? The architect needs a surveyor to bring her expertise—the quality of land needs to be examined, its proneness to flooding assessed, and any legal issues considered. In the analogy, both parties are experts and combine to be effective. To extend the analogy somewhat, the builders are the client's beliefs put into practice and their resources (e.g. social network, finances, coping strategies) the raw materials for construction.

Therapist as a private detective

In the first instance, the therapist needs to gather information. Later, in collaboration with the client, this information needs to be studied to form a coherent story. This facet of CBT has often been likened to a detective's search for evidence. The client often comes for therapy because their life represents an unsolved problem, and the therapist uses questioning to help them find the information that helps to "solve" the problem. Clearly, detectives vary in their interpersonal style, and we would not want to suggest an approach analogous to being grilled by the professionals or being scrutinized within a hard-boiled film noir! The detective of choice for CBT therapists appears to be Columbo, from the long-running American TV series, quiet, curious, unassuming, and even naïve, whether knowingly or otherwise. This approach seems to sidestep his interviewees' defenses and allow them to be more transparent; they know he will not threaten them emotionally or physically in any way. Yet, through the information he gains in this way, the insight to the story behind the crime becomes evident. So, taking this analogy, the way to find out information from our clients is to know that you don't know most of what they have to say, yet have the patience and humility to enquire so that the picture becomes clearer with time. We have found the image of Columbo to help when reviewing therapy during supervision—did you feel that you were being truly open-minded to the client's understanding during the last session? What questions would you ask if you were being truly naïve about what this situation meant to the client? Basically, how would Columbo do it?

Therapist as a coach

This metaphor has made the transition to general usage in the field of "life coaching." However, the popular image of a tracksuit-clad sports coach provides more potent visual content. What is it about coaching that is similar to therapy? First, the coach cannot go out and win the tennis match—this is what the player being coached must do for herself—similarly, in therapy, only the client can live their own life; the therapist will always be one step removed from the "action." Second, coaching is about helping you develop your own strengths and performance on the pitch. What works for you is not the same as what works for the coach: you may have a great capacity for heading a football, but your coach may be a great left-footer. In therapy, the client learns to develop their strengths to deal with their problems with the support of the therapist. Note that the coach is sensitive to the reactions and feedback of the person being coached, just like in therapy. This analogy can be useful when clients feel that only someone who has been through what they have been through can help them; indeed many of the best coaches were not star players themselves, yet they manage to help bring out the best in their players. By a similar token, it can be useful to dispel any idea that one must be "mad" to see a therapist. Serious, very fit athletes and sportspeople usually work with a coach, as do people who are unfit and starting an exercise programme at the gym. Overall, there is much of value in the coach metaphor, although one note of caution perhaps is pertinent: portraying life as a competitive game could be unhelpful for some clients, and therapists should be careful to address any such unintended inference.

Client as a scientist

Behavioural experiments are a cornerstone of cognitive therapy (Bennett-Levy, Butler, Fennell et al., 2004). The fundamental principle is to test a cognition by behavioural means. The modality is an interesting one, as it propels the client into the role of scientist. The therapist is project supervisor, or mentor, and can aid in the careful setting up of the experiment so it tests the right cognitions, under the right conditions, and can assist in interpretation of the outcomes. The "lab" can be many places—the therapist's office, the staircase or lift, the high street, a local shop or café, as appropriate. This metaphorical framework can encourage a spirit of exploration and discovery, essential if clients are to learn more about their world.

Going to the post office

This simple metaphor can provide an antidote to the view that therapy is simply about encouragement, positive thinking, direction by the therapist, and "pushing" the client to do better in some way. It can also help explain resistance and is worth remembering as a therapist. Imagine walking to the post office by yourself. Once you have pictured this, imagine walking to the post office again, but this time with me pushing my finger in your back all the way there, steering you towards it. How would you feel about this? Would you be happy with it, or would you want to push back? What's the problem with me pushing you if I am taking you in exactly the right direction? It seems that even if advice or direction is useful, we want to do things ourselves. And we almost have an instinct to resist a suggestion even if it is the right thing to do. This may explain why for certain clients, the solution to their problems may seem obvious to the therapist, but merely telling them what to do does not work and is met with resistance. It seems to be a universal law of human behaviour— attempts to control other people are met with countercontrol—the explanation is not readily available within CBT theory but may be explained by theories of control such as perceptual control theory (Carey & Bourbon, 2006).

Therapist as a business consultant

This is more appropriate for clients with the experience of business. If the mind is seen as an organization, then the therapist is analogous to a consultant who comes into the organization to help them restructure and become more efficient. The consultant does not run the firm, even temporarily. Their job is to examine its workings and make recommendations, but it is up to the heads of the firm whether they follow these or not. Equally the therapist does not direct the client or tell them what to do. She asks questions to try understand how the client's mind works and how they live their life. She may then make some suggestions that are up to the client to try out for themselves. The idea of the mind as an organization may actually be more that metaphorical. Several psychological frameworks have utilized a hierarchical organization of mental processes in their explanations (Conway & Pleydell-Pearce, 2000; Minsky, 1987; Powers, 1973, 2005). Powers (1973) talks about how effective "reorganization" is responsible for lasting change and recovery within psychological disorders (see also Carey, 2006; Mansell, 2000).

Therapy as a dress rehearsal

The idea of the therapeutic relationship as a potential model for the real world is one that rings true with CBT—role-plays and behavioural experiments both facilitate practice for the outside world through simulation, feedback, and modification, without the same level of risk. This "simulation" metaphor can could come in many guises that would be pertinent to different clients: a miniature model of a new town plan; a flight simulator before piloting a real jet aircraft; a dress rehearsal before the big performance. It is important for therapists to be aware of this inevitability too—how they interact with their clients provides a potential exemplar for their relationships outside the session and vice versa.

Facets of other relationships

Sometimes metaphors are not developed within vastly different domains. They come from links that are drawn between closely related concepts. In the attempt to explain the therapeutic relationship, we find that therapists and clients draw on all kinds of semiformed analogies. Is a therapist like a special kind of friend who listens to you and cares about you, but you don't have to do it in return? Can the therapist act as the nonjudgemental and supporting witness who was not there at the time of a trauma but can be there as you relive the experience? Is she like a biographer, interviewing the client to get all the juicy details, but will never gain financially from knowing all about you? There may be no single answer to these questions, but they provide a way to discuss the nature of relationships and help develop an awareness that they can change over time and can serve different functions depending on the situation. This ability to think flexibly about relationships may be a useful skill we can cultivate in our clients.

Is therapy unique?

We have illustrated a range of metaphors here that illustrate some aspects of the relationship in CBT. We also need to do justice to the reality. The therapeutic relationship is unique in its combination of interpersonal qualities, its guaranteed privacy, and its goal of enhancing mental health in an asymmetrical fashion. Preexisting unhelpful assumptions or fears about the relationship may yield to more helpful yet partly inaccurate mental models, which in turn yield to a less clouded perception of the relationship as a multifaceted and distinctive experience.

Personal responsibility for change

Arguably, when a client signs up for therapy, they are implicitly aware that they are at least superficially demonstrating their responsibility to change in some way. Nevertheless, in practice, willingness to change is not constant, and many people who therapists make contact with have not made this commitment: family members of clients; clients referred by services because of issues of risk to themselves; or others. Even when a person expresses a willingness for *some* kind of change, the therapist cannot assume by how much or in what areas of their life. Certain methods, such as motivational interviewing (Miller and

Rollnick, 2002), are designed to address ambivalence of this kind. There are also metaphors that ring true with certain clients to illustrate and elaborate on the idea of personal responsibility.

Car insurance

It is very likely that some of the causes of psychological problems lie with other people, in what they have done to the client or what they have failed to do in the past, or right now. So, it is very acceptable for our clients to ask why they should have to be the one who has to pick up the pieces and take responsibility for change. It is a very understandable response. The car insurance metaphor provides a familiar way to look at this issue (see also Chapter 12, p. 217). Imagine you are driving a car and someone else bumps into you, damaging your car. Who is to blame? Obviously the other person and his or her insurance will pay for the damage. But who has to contact the insurance company, drive the car to the garage, and check that it has been repaired? You do. In this example, even when another person is completely responsible, we accept that we will have to do something too. This metaphor is unlikely to transform a resistant client instantly, but it provides a common sense example of how we can take responsibility for change even when we are not to blame for the problem.

Health vs illness

Another metaphor along the theme of personal responsibility is more close to home and involves physical illnesses. Many people think that the National Health Service is responsible for "health." Is this right? Surely it is more accurate to say that "illness" is the responsibility of the NHS. Are "illness" and "health" the same thing? It is possible to show that they are two different things because you can be ill and healthy at the same time. The athlete Kelly Holmes is healthy, yet she could still get a cold, she could break a leg, she could get pneumonia. If you became ill what would you do? If you have pneumonia, you may go to the doctor. But if you went to the doctor and said you wanted to be more healthy, what would she tell you? Could she prescribe health? No. She could provide advice about a healthy lifestyle, but this is principally the client's own responsibility to maintain. The same argument can apply to psychological health. Our clients have a responsibility to maintain their own *mental* health; all we can do is help them to work out how to do this most effectively.

Brushing teeth

The idea of change can sometimes feel overwhelming and unfamiliar. But people often fail to see that they experience change all the time in their lives to which they accommodate quite effortlessly. In this therapy dialogue, the example of brushing one's teeth with a different hand was used to develop this idea:

Therapist: Learning to do something differently or something new can be a bit like brushing your teeth with your left hand (if you're right-handed). Unlike the way you normally brush your teeth, which is so automatic you don't even think about it, changing hands feels odd and somehow wrong, and you do it very consciously and perhaps clumsily at first. Have you ever tried it?

Client: Yes, I have once. It was weird, and I kept on missing!

Therapist: What do you think would happen over time if you kept on using your left hand?

Client: I'm not sure, but I guess it would begin to feel "normal."

Therapist: Is there anything inherently bad about brushing your teeth with the "wrong" hand?

Client: Well, no.

Therapist: So just because something feels "wrong" like this doesn't mean that it is wrong, and after time it might begin to feel normal and ok?

Client: Yes, I see. Are you saying that when I get used to behaving differently around other people, I'll get used to it eventually?

Therapist: Well, it's possible, if it's like the brushing example. The way to find out is to try it out a few times I guess?

Client: I can see what you mean. It's probably worth trying.

This is another example of a metaphor in which the content can vary and could be developed from the client's experience: Have you ever tried doing some everyday behaviour in a different way from usual like something you do around the house or at work?

Formulation

A key principle of CBT is the formulation, which is a word that means little to most people. The therapist could simply start drawing the formulation as a diagram and hope that the client gets the idea. A little preamble about what is the function of the shared formulation is clearly recommended, and it is common to use metaphors for this purpose. Very commonly, the formulation is described as a "map" of the problem. This communicates the notion that the formulation is a representation of the problem that is on paper and can be shared and communicated. In a sense, this analogy extends further and relates to the idea of dual expertise between the therapist and the client. Imagine that you had gone for a walk in the local park and you wanted to explain the layout

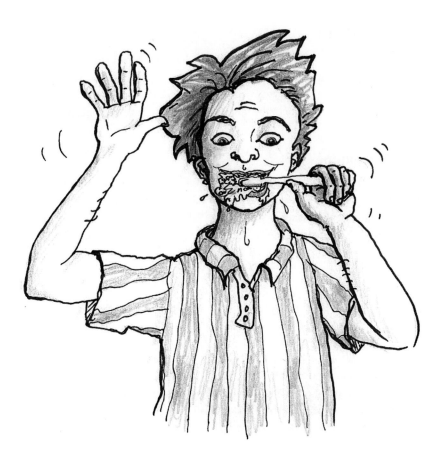

of the park. You could simply explain the layout, but how would we both know that we share the same view. Through drawing out the main landmarks on a map—bandstand, swings, duckpond—and their location with respect to one another, we can be more sure that I have a similar experience of the park as you. The therapist brings the skills of how to draw this "psychological map," but the process is meaningless without the information from the client to complete it. The map analogy is one that can be extended quite readily. We can talk of "looking at it from a new angle," "taking a new route," or "extending the territory." What a map lacks is the sense of change and dynamics that comes from a cognitive formulation. If clients are familiar with flow charts or computer models, they could be introduced. Yet, as mentioned for the therapeutic relationship, metaphors are often only needed as levers or temporary structures, until the concept is experienced in itself and utilized.

Thinking styles

People are often aware that CBT involves "changing how I think," but what exactly does this mean? Without much further elaboration, this idea can become self-evident and even vacuous: "I need to stopping thinking bad things." With the use of metaphor, the role of thinking style can become more tangible.

Simple examples

There are many examples of metaphor to illustrate how people can make interpretations of the same event. Perhaps the simplest and most widespread is the idea that an optimist sees a glass as half full, whereas a pessimist sees a glass as half empty. The fact that this metaphor is so well-known may make it immediately accessible, and yet the therapist and client can still explore it together. Which of these are you—the optimist or the pessimist? Does it depend on the situation, or on how you feel at the time? When do you find it easier to consider both the good and bad points of a situation? What do you make of the fact that a person can think two very different things about exactly the same object? What does this tell us about thinking? These explorations can free up clients to talk about their thinking styles, their context and function, and make attempts at taking different perspectives. On the negative side, simple metaphors of this kind can send out oversimplistic, misleading messages, which the therapist needs to look out for. We are not trying to make our clients "think positively" about every situation; we wish to help them consider multiple perspectives and increase their cognitive flexibility. Thus, gentle probing about what meaning the client is extracting from a metaphor is important, and part of an ongoing process of understanding our client's mental models and how they may change over time.

There are further, richer examples of metaphors to illustrate different interpretations you may wish to read about, including Paul Salkovskis's colourful dog mess story, (Salkovskis, 1996, pp. 48–49; Chapter 3, p. 36) and the well-known burglar metaphor (Beck et al., 1979). In this latter example, a person at home alone one night hears a crash in another room. If their initial interpretation is "There's a burglar in the house" the emotional response is likely to be anxiety. If, however, the interpretation is "Someone left the window open" then the emotional response might instead be annoyance (that one of the kids left it open) or sadness (that something might be broken) (see also Blenkiron, 2005). David Burns uses the example of reading his grade of "D" and immediately assuming it reflects a poor mark rather than the actual meaning—"D" for Distinction (Burns, 1980). Again, the example you choose to use will depend on your own preferences, your client, and the current context. In each case, the metaphor has the capacity to normalize the tendency for all of us to initially jump to conclusions about the meaning of an event, and yet each provides an illustration of how this initial meaning can be captured and an alternative perspective taken.

The filter

The filter idea takes the differing perspectives analogy a step further, and helps to illustrate how a person can take control over the way they frame their experiences. This particular metaphor was developed collaboratively between Helen Morey and one of her clients (see also Chapter 6, p. 115). They came to the view that the brain can be regarded as a "camera," collecting information from the world around it. A person's mood state acts as a "filter" over the camera lens—this makes some aspects of the world appear more vivid (failures, difficulties, etc), whereas other aspects are "washed out and disappear." Within this metaphor, CBT has several related aims. First, it helps people to realize that they are looking at the world through a certain type of filter, in a similar way to the simple examples described earlier. Second, it helps clients to consider that a filter is not fixed but under their control; as they image replacing the filter in their mind's eye, they can prepare for how they might shift their thoughts about difficult situations. Finally, these terms can be used to introduce behavioural experiments assessing the effects of different thinking styles; they can explore the impact of placing different "filters" over the lens on their mood and behaviour.

The black hole

We have included this metaphor as an example of how you can use very vivid and scientific metaphors with some clients. Aidan Bucknall explained to us how he has a particular metaphor he uses with people who have stringent and strong or core belief schemas that are difficult to rate because of their rigidity. It is based on the behaviour of a black hole when a satellite passes a certain point, called the event horizon. An object that passes outside the event horizon continues on its own path but an object that crosses the event horizon is inevitably drawn by gravity to the centre of the black hole. A whirlpool is a more accessible example of the same process; another example can be provided by imagining a marble traveling across a surface that is pulled down at the centre into the shape of a cone. These images are used as metaphors to explain how very strongly held beliefs such as "I am unlovable" draw in one's experiences towards them; they get sucked in. So one day you walk down the street and then someone looks at you and then looks away. If you have this kind of "black hole thinking" then this event comes into your event horizon. Eventually your mind will start reinterpreting the situation: "Why did the person look at me in that way? Because they think I am unlovable." So "I am unlovable" is automatically activated like a thing that gets sucked into a black hole when in the event horizon. The metaphor can help clients visualize and conceptualize the nature of core beliefs, and how they interact with everyday experiences to generate unhelpful automatic thoughts. Like other metaphors, it can now be adapted by clients to help them change their thought processes. The client can identify when the "black hole thinking" occurs. Knowing this the client might opt to change their strategy and think of where the satellite might end up if there was no black hole: What might I be thinking about this experience were I not to have this core belief?

Fawlty towers

Anyone familiar with this enduring comedy will remember that nearly every episode involved Basil, the hotel proprietor, drawing extreme conclusions about his guests and employees that led to bouts of bizarre but comical behaviour.

He tends to act on the ideas that disturb him most without questioning his first impression. For example, in one episode, he tries to catch his guests involved in what he regards as immoral sexual behaviour, yet while this is a misunderstanding on his part, his attempts to try to catch them get him into trouble. In another, he becomes so convinced that a regular guest is a hotel inspector that this leads him to ignore his own rude behaviour towards the real hotel inspector. The most popularly cited episode, *The Germans*, is a tour de force example of the paradoxical effects of thought suppression. Basil tries so hard to not offend his German guests, that his attempts to try to cover his occasional intrusions lead to yet more offensive material that he seems unable to control. Excerpts of *Fawlty Towers* have been used in CBT groups to illustrate concepts such as jumping to conclusions and paradoxical effects of thought suppression and other safety behaviours. Their humour, familiarity, and excessiveness can make these principles highly accessible and clients often feel safer discussing how they affect a third person before they identify them within themselves. While we have highlighted this one comedy series as an example, we are sure that you may have your own favourite. The key is that, like any metaphor, they are used sensitively, within an identified strategy of illustrating an important concept within CBT that could help the client, and that the clients are involved in sharing and discussing their own understanding of the clip.

Pink elephant

There is an overarching principle of CBT that emerges from the realization that thinking styles are flexible. If thoughts really are very flexible, then they can also be arbitrary: what one believes can be independent from reality. This stands in direct contrast to people's typical assumptions before they make this realization: that their thoughts are a direct reflection of reality. In Chapter 5, we will explore metaphors of this kind in more detail as the principle overlaps with the idea of cognitive fusion, developed within the framework of acceptance and commitment therapy (ACT). For now, a metaphor that has appeared in a number of sources provides a nice illustration. If I told you ten times every day that you are a pink elephant, what impact might that have on your beliefs about yourself? Would you start to believe it? If so, would that make you a pink elephant? Is there a difference between your belief and the fact of the situation? This metaphor can then be extended and explored with the client: Are there things that you tell yourself every day? If I told myself that I was useless everyday, would I start to believe it? But would this make it true? Often clients can start to identify their own self-talk and how it colours their view of themselves.

Vicious cycles

Very often, a client's formulation can be represented as one or more "vicious cycles." In other words, the therapist and client discover that the things that the client is doing to try to solve their problem is actually making the problem worse. Often this becomes self-evident. A very common metaphor that seems to emerge from this stage, from both clients and therapists, is "digging to get out

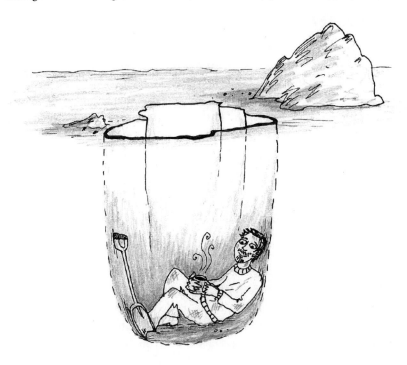

of a hole." The hole represents their problems, and their frantic digging only makes the hole deeper, and more difficult to escape. What is the solution? Shouldn't they do *something* to try to solve their problems even if it doesn't seem to work? In this scenario, the therapist can come back to the metaphor: in this situation, would you continue digging? The answer often seems clearer with this concrete scenario—to *stop* digging, drop the spade and think of some alternative strategies, such as waiting for help, shouting out, clambering out, as long as it is something different. The vicious cycle is a powerful heuristic within CBT yet one that seems to benefit from being grounded within a vivid scenario.

Hayes et al. (1999) describe a nice extension to this metaphor in their ACT approach. To get out of the hole, one needs a ladder. However, one can only hold onto the rungs of the ladder if one lets go of the shovel. Breaking out of vicious cycles of behaviour may require a conscious effort to let go (literally, within the metaphor) of old patterns, which may die hard. To facilitate the utilization of this metaphor, Otto (2000) describes how they used printed cards for clients with shovel and ladder icons on each side. When maladaptive behaviours were identified with clients, they were written onto the "shovel" side along with any associated cues, and behaviours that were agreed as being more helpful were written on the "ladder" side. This represents a creative example of how to maximize the impact and reach of a metaphor beyond the therapy room.

Format of CBT

There are several common components of a course of CBT that can be explained through the use of metaphor. In this section we will cover assessment, the course of therapy, homework, ending therapy, and relapse prevention. Indeed, the use of terms like "homework" and "relapse" prompts images that may be less than desirable, and not truly accurate. Metaphors can help to develop a shared meaning of these components that counters these sometimes confusing or negative connotations.

Assessment

The assessment within CBT is critical, but can be frustrating for some clients who are looking for a "quick fix" to their problems: if they just describe their symptoms then surely the therapist will have some helpful recommendations? Often this belief is based on the model of how their doctor relates to them within a general physician (GP) setting. But as CBT therapists we are aware that this is not sufficient. Not only do we need to understand what is behind our clients' difficulties in more detail, but our approach is to facilitate our client's own perspective and to help them solve their own problems. Helen Morey has tackled this concern by helping clients expand on the medical analogy that they may already use: a psychological assessment is seen as analogous to a full medical examination. In practice, a doctor would not typically prescribe a medication based upon the description of symptoms: she would want to know the reasons for a headache (is it stress, a tumor, the person wearing the wrong glasses, did they hit their head?) beforehand. This requires further, more in-depth examination. Psychological assessment then becomes the equivalent of blood tests, X-rays and such like, rather than equivalent to a superficial discussion with a GP. For some clients, psychological assessments, such as questionnaires may still present difficulties: Does completing these questionnaires say that the client should implicitly be saying "yes" to each of them? The questionnaire can be reframed as an exploratory test. For example, some medical clients cannot describe where or what their symptoms are. In this case, a doctor would likely carry out a physical examination by pressing or bending different parts to see where a reaction occurred. Most people will be familiar with having had this kind of examination at some point in their lives. When this analogy was used, one client then subsequently viewed her self-report scales as "prodding me to see where it hurts," without any assumption that it did (or indeed *should*) hurt where the therapist was "prodding."

The course of therapy

Maybe one of the most important messages to convey for any kind of psychological therapy is that it is not a short-term solution. Change can happen, but it typically happens over a period of time and will involve approaching life goals on a long-term basis. There are some simple analogies for this idea. For example, itching a rash can provide short-term relief and seem like it works for a while, but does it deal with the real cause? Another example that can be particularly pertinent is giving into "the bully." If you were at school and a bully threatened to hit you unless you gave him your dinner money, what would you do? If you gave him your money on Monday, what would he say to you on Tuesday and Wednesday? Would he be more or less likely to take your money in the future? Clients can often identify with a part of themselves that makes threats and that they "give in to," whether it be a worrying thought, a self-critical statement or an obsessive impulse. Therapy is about learning new ways to deal with the bully that do not only involve giving into his demands straight away (see also Chapter 6, p. 122).

Journeys to travel, mountains to climb

Metaphors that see unfolding processes as "journeys" are fundamental in our language. Journeys are not just about literally travelling from A to B. Metaphorically they may represent such varied endeavours as the learning of a musical instrument, the overcoming of a life-threatening illness, the stages of campaigning required to become elected president of the United States, even the stages of life itself "from cradle to grave." Another, closely related form is having a "mountain to climb." Perhaps here there is the added implication of the goal being distant, overwhelming at times, requiring of bravery, persistence, and stamina to succeed. Indeed, so well-worn are the metaphors of the journey and the mountain that they are in danger of becoming clichéd; for example, "the journey of a thousand miles begins with a single step...." However, the process of recovery from psychological problems or disorders is indeed an unfolding, multistage process, and it is not uncommon for clients either to use metaphors such as these or need some guidance as to what to expect through the process of cognitive therapy and beyond. Therefore, as a cognitive therapist, it is worth being able to maximize the usefulness of these metaphors.

For example, the therapist could be the mountain guide. The therapist is the expert in the mountain, but the client knows themselves better than anyone. They can collaborate, discuss pros and cons of different routes up the mountain, explore the territory, and learn more about the mountain, and about themselves. Ultimately it is the client's choice to venture on this expedition; it is their goal, not that of the guide, but the guide will be supportive and point to the client in the right direction to take if they falter. The routes can be steep in places, and there are always ups and downs. Sometimes parts of the journey can feel disheartening, but even setbacks can be useful to learn more about how the mountain works and the guide will help them to get back on their journey. Therapists can be hugely creative in the way such metaphors are used, and with some clients the ideas can be most valuably explored collaboratively, rather than "prescribed." Such a metaphor can offer both orientation and optimism and, assuming it "bites," is then set in place to be referred back to whenever a reminder may be needed.

Not only do such journey metaphors immediately capture the long-term aspect of therapy, but they provide a complexity that lends itself to diverse features of CBT. For example, the client and therapist need to know where they are starting from—what are the problems to be tackled in therapy? They also need to know where they are going to—what are the therapeutic goals? This lends itself nicely to another concept of goal attainment. One cannot plan a journey by saying "I want to be 200 miles away from Manchester." That person could equally well end up in the North Sea, London, or Glasgow! Goals need to be framed as moving *towards* a specific destination rather than as moving *away* from a problem. On the journey, we need to consider what route we are taking, i.e. what therapeutic techniques are to be used or what subgoals make

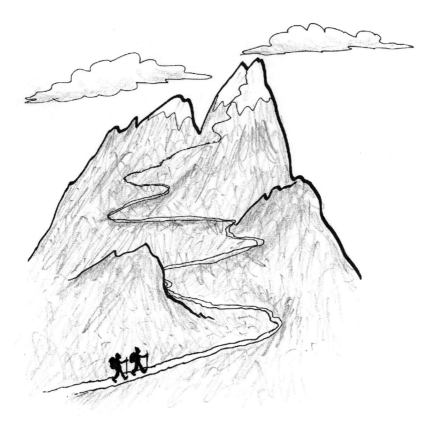

up the overall goal? Features such as the formulation (a map) and contracts (regular breaks in the journey to view the map) can be provided. The therapist works through the map with the client, trying to fathom out a pathway that might get to the destination. In therapy, it is not possible to literally take the client to their destination. This is a journey that the client needs to take for themselves, but the therapist can help them to build up their navigation and map-reading skills.

Ball of string

Another metaphor that illustrates the long-term nature of therapy is provided in a CBT self-help book for coping with fear and phobias (Mansell, 2007) and is reproduced here:

Therapist: Imagine your life is a ball of string, which is lying in an untidy bundle on the floor. The untidy loops and strands are the problems in your life. How would you go about tidying up the ball of string so that you could actually use the string? Would you struggle with the messy loops because you can't tolerate them, yanking the string in different directions? If you were to do this, you would probably make the loops into tight knots that were even more difficult to undo, and you might make the string even messier. Alternatively, would you study the string carefully to see where it was looped round on itself, and then gradually feed through the string so that it could be wound up neatly? This would take a lot longer, but the end product would be simpler and more useful.

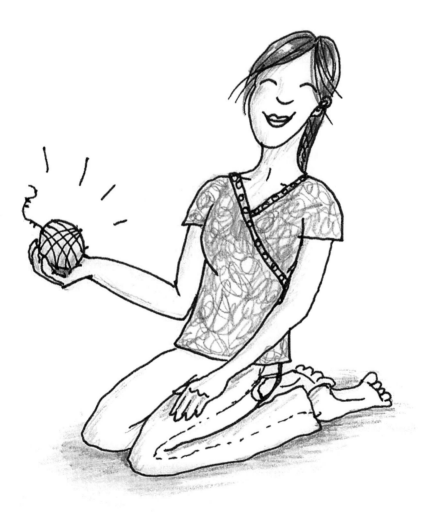

This analogy tries to show that it is possible that we can make our lives more difficult and complex by struggling too hard. On the other hand, if we were to study our experiences, try to understand them, and then apply some strategies that seem to work, this can be more helpful in the long run. This metaphor attempts to contrast short- and long-term coping in a vivid way, and it also incorporates the paradoxical effect of struggling too hard in the here and now, rather than taking a step back to try to understand one's problems in more detail.

Homework, practice, and relapse prevention

Cognitive behavioural therapies typically rely on people doing exercises outside the session—we have a physical metaphor already—the word "exercise," which suggests that we implicitly expect the mind to require practice to stay healthy in the same way as the body requires a workout to stay fit. Practice occurs between sessions as "homework" and after therapy as "relapse prevention." Each of these words, including "exercise" may have negative undertones to the client, depending on their experience with sports, schoolwork, and such like. A metaphorical understanding of our choice of words can help the therapist to be more sensitive in these instances. For example, when the therapist suggests that there is something the client could do in between sessions, she can check whether this raises concerns and the meaning of the "homework assignment" can be unpacked. This needs to be treated sensitively: metaphors are not used in this situation to persuade people but to consider another interpretation of a situation that may lead them to be more willing or not! As a simple example, a sporting individual who performed badly at school may be more willing to consider doing "homework" when they consider it as "exercise for the mind." Many metaphors for practising CBT techniques can be used: musical instruments, games, cooking, and a range of hobbies. However, they can all have connotations of success versus failure, and be very difficult for people who perceive that they have not succeeded through practising any of these skills. A more fundamental metaphor could be used in this case—that of inertia. Any stationary object takes a lot of effort to start moving, like a parked car or a wheelchair. However, once you are moving, the next push takes less effort. Once you are moving quickly, it takes very little effort to keep going, but you never start moving unless you do the first push. This can make sense for people in terms of maintaining their mental health and preventing relapse; although it is easier to keep going once you're moving, if you stop pushing at all, you may grind to a halt and have to get started again. So, it normalizes the tendency to stop using coping techniques as things get easier over time, yet it helps people understand that occasionally they may get a setback and need to use them again. In this metaphor, a coping strategy is the extra push when you notice that things are starting to get difficult. It can help to address ideas clients may have that they either always need to use their coping strategies or they don't need them at all once they are better. The truth, as often, is the mid ground, and in being flexible: Would you use first gear to accelerate while cruising on a motorway? Would fifth gear get a car moving from a standstill? This metaphor could tap into wider issues that we return to later—regarding the self as a dynamic, rather than a static entity, whose pace of development will vary at different times.

The context of CBT

It appears that several key processes are occuring that make it critically important to consider the context of CBT, not only within the health system, but also within academic research, and within society as a whole. First, CBT is expanding in terms of numbers of individuals trained and available to practice. Second, CBT is branching out into related, but clearly differentiated, schools of thought. Third, the public is becoming increasingly aware of CBT, its principles and practice, through the media, government guidelines, and personal experience. Fourth, society as a whole appears to be changing rapidly, with unquestioned respect for authority giving way to a more equal and collaborative, but also potentially more hostile, relationship with authority figures. This heady mixture of trends and changes has the capacity to either make or break CBT, or possibly transform it into something that people do not call CBT any more. There are many possible "traps" for CBT in the world of people's minds. People may become less aware of what it is, as its many branches diverge and its ideas become "watered down" within accessible formats. They may be less likely to see it as distinct from "common sense" as CBT principles become mainstream, or alternatively many may begin to equate it with the "old guard"—a rigid, sterile, mustachioed, general who cannot adapt his terms and techniques to a changing world. Considering that social evolution is inevitable, maybe it would be beneficial for CBT to embrace this change and allow a transition that maintains what we as therapists value most—the quality of life of fellow beings. Could there be metaphors that help us to see where CBT is now, and where it may go in the future? They would be useful not only for our clients but also for other health professionals, service purchasers, and the general public.

Cognitive behavioural therapies as a family of therapies

Families change over time. People are born, they die, they arrive, and they leave. Relationships are formed and broken. Similarly, CBT has been changing dynamically (for more detail, see Mansell, 2008a, 2008b). It has had a burgeoning band of champions, some of whom are sadly no longer with us. Others have formed their own brand of CBT or "jumped ship" entirely. Collaborations and links between different brands of CBT have been formed (for example between ACT, mindfulness based CBT, and dialectical behaviour therapy). When clients ask "What is CBT?" maybe one answer to this question is that CBT is very much a family of related therapies. This analogy is similar to Wittgenstein's notion of "family resemblances" as a more appropriate way to provide a definition of a concept. Yet the parallels can be made more directly—there are several "related" CBT therapies; some are more closely related than others; the relationship between them is typically positive but in some instances it can be conflictual.

The metaphor can be extended—this CBT family, in turn, has distant relations with other therapies, which can often be important—both for good and bad reasons. In this scenario, maybe classic psychoanalysis is like the colourful but embarrassing uncle who comes for Christmas. Some of the family love him and soak up his wild ideas, others think he is just quirky but harmless, and a few of the family unit just can't stand him! This mixed response from proponents of CBT to other psychological therapies may be familiar. We have heard of one metaphor used to describe CBT: "The Borg" from *Star Trek*: The Next Generation. This is a gigantic, amorphous computerized block that travels through space, absorbing and assimilating everything and everyone around it. In the series, the Borg is one of Captain Picard's most formidable adversaries. It seems as though the tendency for CBT to incorporate principles and techniques from a diverse ranges of therapies can clearly have negative connotations to some people, especially if it does so without due credit or without distinguishing itself from its predecessors in the ancestral line. While these issues surrounding the development of CBT will clearly be around for a while, maybe the family metaphor can give us reason to be hopeful. We know that families are continually undergoing change, past transgressions can be acknowledged and forgiven, and previous conflicts can be turned into constructive, equal relationships given the right circumstances.

The role of CBT within the "medical model"

For many of our clients it is critical to locate the role of CBT, or psychology, or the "mind" in general, within a medical framework. It is through medical services that our clients typically come to see us after all, so surely we have a framework to use to explain this connection? A common approach is to see biological factors either as "risk" factors (e.g. genes), or as processes that have reciprocal relationships with psychological processes. For example, the cognitive model of panic (Clark, 1986) proposes that changes in bodily sensations trigger catastrophic thoughts about those sensations, which in turn activate a fear response which through the sympathetic nervous system evokes a further physiological reaction. This wordy explanation can be aided by a simple diagram, but can metaphors provide a more accessible way to get across this close link between the mind and body; thought and biology; psychology and medicine?

One common example is dealing with a client who is taking medication as well as receiving CBT. Often the choice of both of these interventions seems to send out conflicting messages—one that the problem is physical and the other that it is psychological—and clients struggle with what this means about the causes of their problems. One metaphor regards medication as "bike stabilizers" whereas CBT is the process of learning to ride a bike. Learning to ride a bike is easier with stabilizers. In this respect, medication may help to reduce symptoms somewhat and make it easier to engage in therapy. However, this metaphor makes another matter clear: You do not learn to ride a bike simply by attaching stabilizers to the wheels. Learning is critical, otherwise the stabilizers will always be needed. Hence the aim of CBT is to help the client manage their mind and their life more effectively so that in the future they may be less reliant on medication - the goal is to learn to ride a bike without stabilizers. This metaphor can be richer than it appears. For example, if a client stops taking their medication suddenly as soon as they have a "good day," this can set them back as their symptoms return to them unexpectedly. Within the metaphor, this is explained: if the client was in the early stages of learning to ride a bike and they happened not to fall off one day, would this mean that they are ready to remove the stabilizers? In reality, a person would wait until she could ride the bicycle well, under different conditions, before abandoning the stabilizers for good.

Often clients come with a medical model of their psychological problems, and an alternative understanding seems necessary before they begin to experiment with changing their thinking or their behaviour. For example, they believe that because their feeling of depression is so strong, it is due to a physical cause. This is of course partly true in the immediate term—depression is associated with physical brain changes—so to help these clients to build a role for their thoughts and behaviour in recovery can be challenging. Rather than questioning the client's initial account, it can be powerful to go along with their view and explore exactly what kind of physical problem might be an analogy for what is going on for the client. Many medical conditions are not regarded as severe, isolated, or irreversible. They are either systemic diseases (e.g. heart disease, diabetes) or they represent lesions to these systems from which they naturally recover (e.g. the immune system fights viral infections). In addition, the clinical recommendations for many systemic illnesses are behavioural such as changing diet and exercising as an intervention for heart disease. An example of therapy dialogue will be used here to illustrate how this metaphor can be used in practice:

Client: Sometimes I don't see how just talking to you about my problems can help—it just seems as though my brain has changed permanently.

Therapist: Tell me how you think your brain has changed.

Client: Well it's just like, since I've been depressed, it's like fuzzy, like cotton wool. I think I have damaged it in some way. Something physical has changed – its not just what I am thinking about.

Therapist: So, if it has changed physically, what do you think would help?

Client: Well the medication is designed for that, isn't it? I think my tablets have made it better, a lot more manageable.

Therapist: Right, so one thing that helps is the medication. If you just had the medication, would that be enough?

Client: Not really. I still feel low even on the medication. It takes the edge off I think. I need something more, but I don't know what that is.

Therapist: If it were something physical, what do you think you would need, besides the medication, to help it get better?

Client: What do you mean?

Therapist: Well, if, say it were your heart, and you needed to take medication to lower your cholesterol, that would be a physical problem, right?

Client: Yes, that would definitely be physical.

Therapist: And so, I am thinking if your brain is affected physically, and its similar, what might a person need to do to make a physical organ like the brain or the heart better, when it's not working as well as it should do?

Client: Well I guess someone with a heart condition needs to rest. But then they do say that you need to exercise more, to get it more healthy, like a muscle. Well it is a muscle really.

Therapist: Yes, that's what I was thinking, that a heart needs exercise, and so does a brain, as it's really just another part of the body. I guess that is really what I think we have been trying out in the sessions – exercising your mind, to get it to do what it is designed to do – help you get what you want out of life.

Client: And you think that just by talking about these things, it will change my brain, get rid of this cloudiness I get all the time?

Therapist: Well, we know that when a person has a thought, there are changes in their brain. I don't know what causes the fuzziness you are experiencing, but we could experiment with it. Maybe we could try 'exercising' your brain one day and seeing what the effects are, and we can compare that to a day when you don't exercise it—you can do what you usually do when you feel low that day. What do you think?

Client: Well I guess there is no harm trying. If you are right, and I can make that physical change just by thinking differently then I would want to know about it. I am willing to give it a try.

In this example, the therapist worked partly through Socratic questioning and partly through direct psychoeducation. As mentioned in Chapter 3, the style of presenting metaphors is likely to vary between therapists, between clients, and within the same client on different occasions. Nevertheless, when engaged in questioning it is important to be open-minded about what understanding the client will reach and be flexible enough to use their language and build on their metaphor if it looks promising. Equally, when providing information, it is important to be aware of any assumption you have that the client will respond in a particular way when they are given that information. They will interpret and use that information according to their preexisting beliefs and this may involve dismissing the information completely. Thus, both questioning and psychoeducation have the risk of promoting resistance in the client; yet through respect of the client's self-determination and an attentiveness to their perceptions and interpretations, a shared metaphor is likely to be developed in a collaborative manner.

CBT, protocols, and the surgery metaphor

How many times have we heard the phrase "Client X could do with a bit of CBT"? Is a "bit of CBT" analogous to a "bit of Fluoxetine"? The implicit metaphor here is that CBT can be dispensed in a dose-related manner rather like medicine. Of course, numerous randomized controlled trials have directly compared a form of CBT for a given disorder to a specific medicine, in order to evaluate the relative efficacies of a psychological and a pharmacological approach. But while we may value such research a great deal, and in many cases agree that Client X indeed could benefit from "a bit of CBT"—it is worth reflecting that the implicit metaphor here is rather shaky, in a number of respects. CBT is not a pure, unchanging, decontextualized intervention that is readily compared to a tablet. As mentioned earlier, CBT is really better thought of as a family of related therapies. Indeed, many variables potentially affect what CBT is—the presenting problem(s), the idiosyncrasies of the case, the school of training from which the therapist has come, the level of competence and skill of the therapist, the nature of therapist's supervision, the interpersonal dynamics of the therapist–client dyad, and so on.

A more accurate variant on the medical metaphor might therefore be "CBT as surgery." Indeed, surgery is a skilled endeavour, requiring extensive training and ongoing supervision. It is goal-focussed and seeks to deliver optimal outcomes for clients. It is based on well-developed theories and knowledge of the workings of human beings, and has evolved specific tools and techniques which are evidence-based but which can be carefully tailored to the individual case. Surgery can also, it must be said, be done well or done badly. In many respects, therefore, surgery is conceptually more comparable to CBT than medicine, and helps highlight the important factors of quality and context of delivery of the intervention.

A related extension to the surgery metaphor concerns the issue of protocol-driven approaches to cognitive therapy. One common anxiety among some therapists is that by following a standardized protocol in their approach to a client's problems (e.g. panic disorder) they may be reducing their flexibility and ability to help. However, the surgery metaphor would suggest, on the contrary, that protocols and flexibility are not mutually exclusive, and indeed they can act synergistically. For example, a heart surgeon has "standardized tools" for his job. He knows, specifically, the nature of intervention he needs to undertake, the general principles and procedures that he will follow. But this does not mean he wields his scalpel without regard for the individual presentation or nuances of the case. Indeed, his protocols, tools and well-honed procedures *free him up* and allow him the flexibility to accurately monitor, appraise and adjust his interventions in an optimal manner. He does not have to waste time reinventing the wheel during each operation—thinking about how heart valves might work or what kinds of knives or monitoring instruments might be helpful.

Likewise, in CBT, following a model and a protocol, especially in cases where good results have been reliably researched, can enhance and free up the clinician's ability to think flexibly and to tailor an effective intervention around a coherent set of well-tested principles. This is not to denounce the welcome nature of innovation in therapy, and treatment developments can and do emerge from the clinical setting as much as from the laboratory (see also a discussion of empirically grounded clinical interventions, Chapter 13, p. 229). But perhaps it will be useful for us to remember that heart surgeon when we consider these issues in our therapeutic work.

Summary

Throughout this chapter, we have illustrated how different metaphors can be used to emphasize and explain different facets of the therapeutic relationship in CBT. An essential feature of any psychotherapy is taking personal responsibility for change and the reasons for this can be illustrated using metaphor. In particular, cognitive therapy is about people's "way of thinking"; this is an abstract term that is illuminated through metaphors from simply the idea of a "glass half empty" to more elaborate examples. Furthermore, the way that CBT is structured (e.g. assessment, homework) can be illustrated for the client through metaphor and as CBT practitioners, we can situate the ongoing development of CBT within its scientific and clinical context using metaphors and analogies.

Chapter 5

Conceptualizing cognition and metacognition

Introduction

One of the great contributions of CBT to psychological treatment is its capacity to help characterize cognitions within the individual who presents with distress. Often the term "cognition" is understood to refer to cognitive content such as what a thought "says" ("I have made a complete fool of myself!"). However, this definition of cognition is limited. We take a broad view of "cognition" that includes those concepts studied in the domain of cognitive psychology, including perception, attention, memory, imagery, the process of learning, and the process of managing cognitions themselves (typically known as "metacognition"; Flavell, 1979). This broader definition is critical for several reasons. First, it provides a more comprehensive coverage of what is really going through our clients' minds; the phenomenology of the experience. If we want to try to understand clients from their perspective, this is the stance we need to take and it would seem arbitrary to draw the line at certain phenomena that might not fit a narrow definition of cognition. Second, our approach generally reflects how CBT has developed within the last three decades, as cognitive psychology and CBT have become more closely linked and the processes of attention, memory, and reasoning have become better defined and understood. Most contemporary CBT models explicitly identify these processes (e.g. Clark & Wells, 1995; Garety et al., 2001; Rapee & Heimberg, 1997; Wells, 1997; Ehlers & Clark, 2000). Third, there is a clear debate about the nature of cognition within frameworks such as relational frame theory (RFT; Hayes, 2004), interacting cognitive subsystems (ICS; Teasdale & Barnard, 1993) and perceptual control theory (PCT; Powers, 1973; 2005) and so it would seem prudent to define cognition broadly until a deeper consensus is achieved within the field of CBT.

In this chapter, we wish to share examples of metaphors that illustrate the various facets of cognition in ways that appear therapeutic to clients and may often indicate a shift in their perspectives on their thought processes. We will begin with an overview of how different kinds of processes can be explored and identified using metaphors. Then, we have found that the metaphors used with clients seem to cluster around two themes—the nature of learning and memory and the nature of metacognition, or relationship with one's own cognitions and how to manage them. This area seems to be one where working with the clients' own metaphors is particularly pertinent—after all we are trying to understand the other person's inner mental world, and it would seem most appropriate to do this from the client's own inner perspective on their thoughts.

Exploring and identifying cognitive processes

The client's descriptions of their own perceptions are often metaphorical, possibly because they are trying to communicate about a felt sense that is not directly observable to others. They need metaphors of entities in the outside world to describe them. Simply listening to these metaphors and exploring why they are used can provide a window to the client's inner world, and promote their own, and their therapist's understanding. Some of the memorable metaphors we have encountered relate to the nature of thinking during extreme states such as depression, acute anxiety, and psychosis. We have provided an example here that actually occurred towards the end of therapy, but it illustrates quite how much client-generated metaphors in this area can be brought out to develop a shared understanding between the client and the therapist.

Spaghetti

Therapist: Can you tell me how you think things have changed for you during the therapy so far?

Client: Well, I said before that my mind was like spaghetti, all twisted up, and confused. That's what it was like when I first came to see you.

Therapist: Spaghetti?

Client: Yes, I know it sounds silly, but, let me explain. Spaghetti is gloopy. Is that the word? It's all soggy and moist and it's so knotted that you just can't get it straight. That's what I have been doing—trying to get these strands of spaghetti straightened out. Everyone has some knots in their spaghetti—you can't get rid of all of them. But what we have been doing has helped me get rid of some of these knots.

Therapist: That sounds really visual as you're telling me this. Let me just try to understand this. The spaghetti is your thoughts, right?

Client: Yes, my thoughts were so messed up when I was ill, and I knew it was because of what had happened to me—the traumas we have talked about—and these are the knots.

Therapist: OK, and everyone has some knots?

Client: Yes, you can't go through life without some problems, but I have had more than most people.

Therapist: Yes, and the straightening out?

Client: That's when we have talked about these traumas and I have put them behind me, so I don't need to think about them again. Well I do a bit, but not as much as before.

Therapist: So, why this gloopy—is that what you said?—this gloopiness?

Client: I'm not sure. I felt it wasn't easy, but it was worth it in the end.

Therapist: So, talking about what had happened to you, and all the emotions that came up then, that was getting your fingers messy, taking this strands of spaghetti out, and untying them.

Client: Yes, that's what it felt like. And I know that I'll always have some of these knots but I think my mind is a lot straighter now. Everything is calmer. I am more content.

This example clearly illustrates how clients' metaphors can combine many individual concepts into a single idea. The notion of the mind being like spaghetti could be dismissed easily if the therapist is not listening attentively. However, if the therapist has in mind the goal of elucidating the client's experiences, and gives them the time and space as well as encouragement to reflect on their experiences, fruitful discussions may emerge. Some clients clearly work more naturally with metaphors and use this skill to develop shared understandings with metaphorically minded therapists. This particular client used a large number of them. For example, he worked in a paint factory in which he mixed pigments and solvents in huge vats. At the end of each shift, there was a "residue" of paint that needed to be cleared from the vats to prepare them for the next mix. During therapy he was trying to come to terms with the fact that he had not fully recovered from his last episode of depression—he would still wake up occasionally in very low moods and they would last throughout the day. He was very afraid that they signalled a relapse. The therapist was trying to help him reframe these experiences as a natural consequence of a very distressing time, and talked about the nature of memory in quite concrete terms. The client suddenly grasped this idea, but not through an abstract knowledge of psychology. He saw that these isolated low moods were the "residue" of his depression. When he and his therapist explored the metaphor, they talked about how a residue is an inevitable consequence of a previous paint mix. Although it could contaminate the next paint mix, it generally did not because it was dealt with in a straightforward way—by clearing out the vat. In the same way, low moods and distressing memories are an inevitable consequence of a past series of traumas. They can "contaminate" the day, but they do not need to do so if they are dealt with in an effective way.

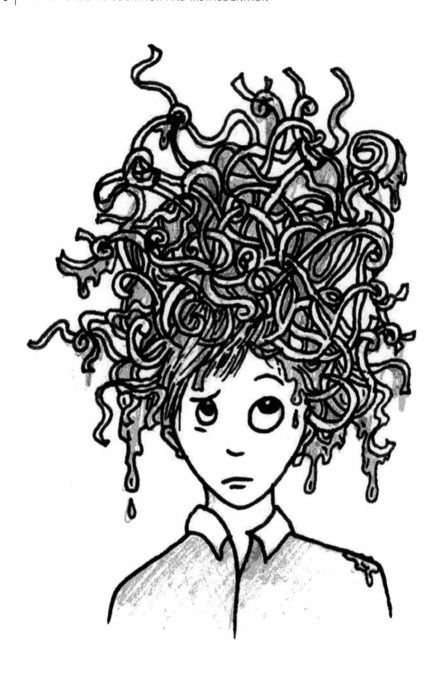

How to develop these effective strategies was the next step, and led on to a discussion of coping strategies to do with acceptance and attentional redirection.

How the mind works

Sometimes, our clients have an unhelpful notion of how the human mind works, yet they are keen to learn more about psychology to update their views. Certain metaphors can help to illustrate these principles, which then have an effect on the expectations that the client has about how their mind should work. In this section we will focus on metaphors that illustrate the reasons why the mind can often be resistant to change, and techniques and principles that can facilitate more productive, long-lasting progress.

Automaticity

Contrary to a popular misconception, cognitive behavioural therapies consider automatic mental processes as important. Indeed, Aaron T. Beck's initial model conceived of negative automatic thoughts (NATs; Beck, 1967). These were conceptualized as fleeting cognitions that may pass through consciousness rapidly with little consideration yet have a huge impact on lowering mood in people with depression. The therapist's goal is first to help the client notice and identify these thoughts before their validity can be challenged or explored using evidence from experience. Much of contemporary CBT, such as mindfulness and metacognitive therapy, also involves helping clients to become more aware of the stream of automatic thoughts in their consciousness. These approaches comply well with current accounts of automatic mental processes within the field of cognitive psychology (Hassin, Uleman, & Bargh, 2005). Nevertheless the notion of automatic processes can be difficult to explain and discuss with clients and therefore everyday examples can make these more accessible.

One metaphor can be targeted towards clients who are computer literate. The "subroutine" idea concerns the processes of cognitive change. It illustrates that "everything we learn we never forget. And, most of what we've learnt, we don't know we've learnt it." It can also be used to illustrate the automaticity of relapse prevention. The metaphor is that you are typing a letter on your computer and you want to underline some text. So, you press the U icon on a word processor. When you select the U icon "you didn't have to type in loads of instructions in order to underline your text." All you had to do was press the U icon. Analogously, when you are home and you want a cup of tea you do not need to think of every step you take in order to make that cup of tea. You probably make the cup of tea and converse with a friend and you do not have to think

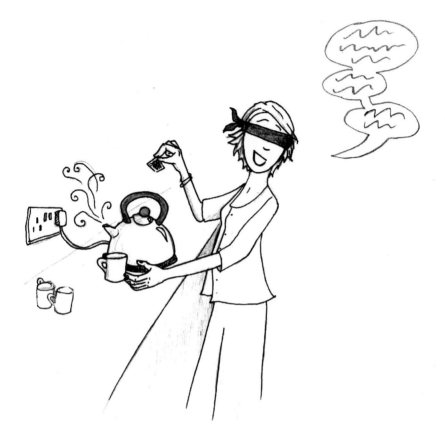

about the steps. The reason for this is that the stages become routine and the routine is embedded. All it requires is a trigger such as "I would like a cup of tea" and there follows a procedure, i.e. make the cup of tea. In the same vein, when you need to change gear in a car, you do not need to tell yourself the exact movements of your legs and arms you need to make. This process has become automatic once learned.

In a similar manner, people often jump over numerous links in their chains of thought. A person may see someone who they know at a party. They go up to talk to them, but this person does not react in the positive way they had imagined. The thought that is automatically activated is "I am going to be alone for the rest of my life." So, none of the links in the chain of thought leading to that conclusion are appraised—the automatic thought dominates because it is routinized. The "subroutines" idea describes this process of jumping the intermediate links between thoughts to arrive at an end (often negative) thought. Therapy is often about identifying these intermediate stages and questioning them through logic and evidence. This may not be enough, how-ever, to help people function better. We might also need to write or re-write new subroutines that work better. They may not be perfect, but they are adapt-able and can be modified. The original routine does not dissipate but rather is replaced and modified. However, there will always be cases and circumstances where the original routines may be activated and the person needs to accept, be mindful of, and prepared for this. Once clients are conscious of this, they can often manage more successfully as they can call on and apply the modified routines.

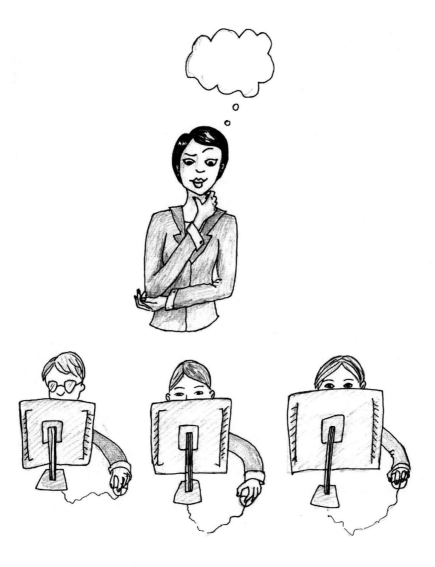

An alternative metaphor is one of managing a company where the boss of the company represents the conscious decision-making process and their employees represent the automatic routines that guide their everyday behaviour. Most of the time, the boss does not need to be involved in the running of the company; his employees manage the functioning of the company. Yet, every so often, issues emerge that cannot be dealt with by others and he needs to consider such issues himself. Often making necessary changes to a large company can be difficult, as it depends on transmitting information down through the organization. In this respect, one can see how awareness may not be involved in habitual activities, yet it is critical for resolving problems that do arise. It also illustrates that while decisions to change can be made by an individual, it may take time for these to "trickle down" to everyday behaviours. The client may need to recall and consider their higher level goals at these times as the rest of the mind may not be ready yet for the changes ahead.

This approach is not only a metaphor, but represents the kind of approach that has been taken to the workings of the mind in theories such as those of Marvin Minsky (1987), William T. Powers (1973), and Selfridge (1959). Another very accessible idea is to see the unconscious mind as an "elephant" that we are riding and trying to steer through our lives (Haidt, 2006). It is not like a car that we can control with ease and flexibility, but has a "mind" of its own, to some extent. This view helps to validate the struggle that people have with their own minds. It may prompt them to realize that the process of change can be slow at times and that it may involve an acceptance of the resistance of their own mental processes to change as well as the learning of new skills to manage these resistant processes.

Emotional responses to change situations

An early response to therapy can involve a fear of change. This is normal and metaphors can be used to demonstrate how everyone may experience such emotional reactions to novel situations. For example, the following everyday analogy can be helpful:

Therapist: Learning to do something differently or something new can be a bit like brushing your teeth with your other hand (see Chapter 4, p. 55). Unlike the way you normally brush your teeth, which is so automatic you don't even think about it, changing hands feels odd and somehow wrong, and you do it very consciously and perhaps clumsily at first.

Client: [discussion with therapist]

Therapist: What do you think would happen over time if you kept on using your left hand?

Client: It would start to feel normal.

Therapist: So, is there anything inherently bad about brushing your teeth with the "wrong" hand?

Client: No.

Therapist: So, maybe just because something feels "wrong" like this doesn't mean that it is wrong, and after time it might begin to feel normal and OK?

This simple analogy may not work with everyone; other examples may help, such as learning to drive on the other side of the road in a different country, or

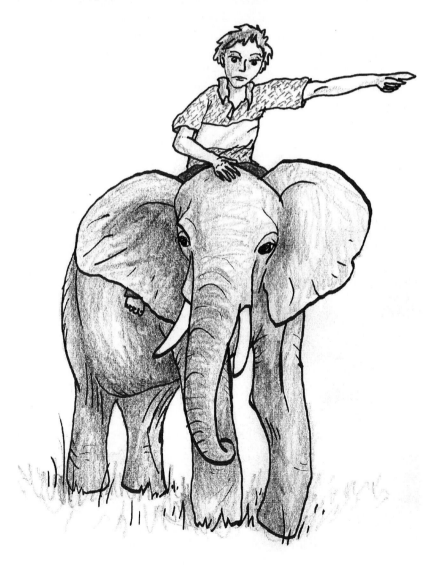

encouraging the client to cast their mind back to a time when they had learned a new skill. In each case, the aim is to help the client to accept their discomfort when confronting change and help them to draw on experiences in which they showed flexibility and built up confidence and skill at a task that had appeared daunting at first.

The importance of practice

An implication of what has been said above is that change requires time. Critically, it is the process of practice over time that helps people to learn new skills or break old habits of thinking. There are a flurry of accessible metaphors to illustrate the importance of practice, the most obvious being sporting performance and mastery of a musical instrument. Other examples can be targeted at the client group involved—for example, the extensive practice that teenagers have with computer games may provide an excellent example of how practice, perseverance and motivation enhance performance. One important slant on the metaphor is to explain how practice is not only helpful, but necessary in some instances where the final "performance' requires an already well-developed skill. If you were learning how to tightrope over the Grand Canyon (which many people have attempted since the Victorian era!), then you would start in a simple, safe way, such as walking over a narrow beam that is a foot above the ground. Next, you might choose to raise the height, or narrow the walkway, but in small steps. It would clearly not only be impossible to achieve the Grand Canyon feat straight away, but very dangerous! Swimming the channel or running a marathon are other patent examples. The strength of the metaphor lies in the clarity of connection that can be made to the client's presenting problem, and its propensity to validate the struggle that the client faces, yet to present them with a slow and steady way of managing it rather than the "boom and bust' approach that they might have used in the past. Practice metaphors can apply to diverse areas that require learning and adaptation, such as recovery from depression, facing fears, changes in interpersonal style, processing of trauma, and learning relapse prevention.

The importance of organization and coherence

Often the acquisition of knowledge and learning of skills can appear to be a process of collection, or even hoarding, of information and experience. While this is clearly part of the process, it is easy to overlook the importance of *organization* of information into a coherent, understandable whole. Often clients are very good at searching for information and advice, but less able to integrate and reflect on this information so that it is usable and relevant to them.

One of the clearest examples is the way in which information is encoded after a trauma or period of multiple traumas. It is often fragmented and incoherent, and therefore not easily consciously accessed and recalled. The felt sense experienced by many clients is that of confusion as they struggle to make sense of their extreme experiences and reconcile their personal meanings. In clients who have experienced psychosis, this sense of confusion may be felt particularly acutely, and they appear to direct their lives towards the desperate pursuit of imposing meaning on confusing inner experiences, some of which may be earlier memories or sensory recollections.

Several everyday metaphors can help to validate this confusion and illustrate the process of recovery through reorganization. In posttraumatic stress disorder (PTSD), there are the "filing cabinet" and "overfull cupboard" metaphors for memory (e.g. Ehlers and Clark, 2000; see also Chapter 7, p. 151). Trauma memories are like loose files in a disorganized office, scattered around different cabinets, often turning up under your nose when you don't expect them. Recovery from trauma is like going through these memories one at time and inspecting them to work out where to file them. "Did I experience this before or after the accident?"; "I had this feeling that other people were present during the trauma—by processing the memory I now remember who these people were." In this way, the client can now start to organize her memories into a coherent narrative in a chronological order, like a well-ordered filing cabinet going from A to Z. The overfull cupboard analogy is similar; in this one the overwhelming nature of a traumatic memory is also captured by the vivid spectacle of a hurriedly stuffed cupboard bursting open with all its contents spilling out. The solution—to spend time processing and reorganizing the contents of the cupboard. It may become clear to both client and therapist that nearly every complex system has an ordered structure—the folder structure on a computer; the hierarchy of a company; the chapter structure of a book—and that given the enormous amount of information within memory, the necessity of organization becomes obvious. Perhaps in the broadest sense, provision of the space, and tools for clients to begin to make sense and order out of the chaos of their lives is a goal of all therapies.

Negative automatic thoughts and dysfunctional attitudes

Moving into more traditional CBT territory, we may benefit from developing analogies to communicate the ideas of "negative automatic thoughts" (or NATs), "dysfunctional assumptions," and "core beliefs" (see also Chapter 6, p. 110). Therapists are likely to vary in their desire to educate their clients in their use of these terms. Nevertheless, their essence can be important to distil—NATs sweep fleetingly though consciousness whereas dysfunctional assumptions are deeply held personal rules about how to live one's life, and core beliefs the foundations through which all experiences are filtered. The latter two of these, the "schematic" components of our cognitive frameworks, we may be particularly unaware of on a conscious level. Often these terms are best introduced as "thoughts," "rules," and the "bottom line" (Fennell, 1999) as they arise in the therapeutic dialogue rather than invoking their technical wording. A helpful analogy we have encountered is used in the computerized CBT package, *Beating the Blues*™ (Proudfoot et al., 2003), but is likely to have much earlier origins. NATs are likened to leaves of a tree and dysfunctional assumptions and core beliefs (or schemas) as the roots of the tree. This encapsulates the relatedness of the thoughts and assumptions and core beliefs while illustrating their differences. Like leaves sweeping through a breeze, NATs are briefly conscious thoughts that pass through awareness. Like the roots, personal rules, assumptions, and core beliefs are more permanent and are more difficult to access, yet they feed the thoughts much like roots feed nutrients to the tree. The metaphor can make the difficulty of challenging long-held personal rules and core beliefs become clearer—it may feel like removing the foundations of one's thoughts and feelings. Maybe an alternative is to build new growths to alternative sources before taking the risk of allowing familiar roots to wither? This extension of the metaphor fits well with the clinical reality of helping clients to balance the building of support mechanisms, coping strategies, and personal beliefs with the challenging of existing thoughts and assumptions.

Separation of rational and emotional

Very often clients notice a discrepancy between what they believe at a rational level and what they *feel* to be true when they are emotional. Sometimes they will state the *"feeling as if"* belief (e.g. *"it feels like the roads are just too dangerous"*) and go on to say "But I know it's irrational!" Other times clients will do the reverse; they will provide rather a logical and intellectual answer to a question about how something felt to them. None of this, of course, is their fault. Our minds are complex, and our commonplace language of "belief" and "knowing" sometimes does a mediocre job of describing the multiple streams of rational and irrational cognition, which battle for attention inside our heads. Sometimes, these discrepancies can be the source of much frustration, and even thoughts that they are going mad. Hence, a person with a lift phobia may clutch their head in dismay, declaring "I know it's safe!" A woman with PTSD who was raped knows rationally that lying down is perfectly safe, but is infuriated by experiencing fear and vulnerability when she does so, as if something terrible will happen again. Teasdale and Barnard (1993) have previously suggested introducing the terminology of "intellectual belief" and "emotional belief" to characterize these processes, and others have examined this phenomenon of rational-emotional dissociation extensively (Stott, 2007).

To help clients make sense of these issues it can be helpful to utilize the meta-phorical language of "divided parts of the self." There are various terminologies to achieve this; multiple armies battling for attention is one possibility, multiple "voices" is another (see also Chapter 6, p. 122). Consider the following dialogue between the therapist and the client (who has previously suffered a road traffic accident).

Therapist: So how did it feel when you walked down the high street?
Client: Well, it's really stupid, because I know it's completely safe, hundreds of people go there every day and they're fine.
Therapist: OK, so that may be true, but that sounds like the rational, logical bit of you saying that. If we leave the logical bit to one side for a moment, I was wondering what it felt like?
Client: Not good. I felt kind of horrible, like I wanted to get out of there.
Therapist: And what was your worst fear, when you were there?
Client: Well, like I say, I didn't really believe anything could happen, to be honest—I don't think there was anything to fear really—it's just a completely average, normal place, and it was just an average, rainy day, that's the ridiculous thing.
Therapist: Yes, but I guess that sounds like the rational voice piping up again? Just remembering back to that feeling you had, walking down there on that rainy day, what did it *feel* like might happen—even if it doesn't seem to make much logical sense?
Client: It felt like a car might suddenly mount the pavement and hit me.
Therapist: Might mount the pavement and hit you?
Client: Yes.
Therapist: That sounds like a terrifying feeling.
Client: Yep. But that's crazy isn't it?
Therapist: Well, the rational part inside you might not think it made much sense, but the feeling part was very powerful and very real by the sound of it.
Client: Yes it was scary, and I get that whenever I go out. That's why I hate going out.
Therapist: OK, so if I've understood you right, it sounds like there's a rational voice which is telling you the cars and pavements are safe, but then there's an emotional voice which keeps telling you that "those cars are dangerous and might mount the pavement any minute". Is that right?
Client: Exactly.

Selective processing

A number of cognitive biases are seen across a wide range of disorders, and metaphors may be needed to help explain to clients the cognitive processes in question (Harvey, Watkins, Mansell, & Shafran, 2004). For example, the common process of selective attention could be likened to a "spotlight." Your attention is a spotlight, and hence it gets focused on one thing. You miss out on other things because the spotlight keeps getting drawn to one part of the situation (the negative part) like a magnet. The goal is to "broaden" the spotlight—to see the whole situation in a real and unbiased manner (see also Chapter 7, p. 132 for a more detailed look at selective attention in the context of anxiety).

Another selective process is that of selective memory for events. A straightforward, normalizing, and broadly applicable analogy here is that of a commonplace experience—trying to remember a song and only being able to recall the chorus. One has a "selective memory" for the most prominent part of the song.

Expectancy biases are also common across disorders, and a personal example from Roz Shafran demonstrates one such expectancy bias rather nicely (Harvey et al., 2004). While writing her thesis, she was nervous about the first chapter she handed in and which she believed was rubbish. When the manuscript returned, the comment was "I've stopped reading for the writing style from hell." Only on a calmer re-reading did she discover that the comment actually read "I've stopped reading for the writing style from here." Her negative prediction of criticism had influenced her perception of events.

Recurrent thinking

Recurrent thinking, such as rumination or worry, is another common cognitive process across disorders (Harvey et al., 2004). At the simplest level, the therapist might want to normalize this process. Recurrent thinking is like when you've had an argument with someone. You know the process? The contents of the argument go round and round and you replay the argument, thinking of all the other things you could have said. The client might be asked whether they recall this ever happening to them—invariably the answer is yes. See p. 94 for a further discussion of recurrent thinking, and also Chapter 6 (p. 119) for a more detailed look at rumination in the context of depression.

Use of movies

Within this area, we have become aware of several popular movies that vividly illustrate cognitive behavioural processes. They are perhaps more useful in illustrating the processes during the training of therapists rather than with clients during therapy. For example, the movie *Adaptation* begins with a blank screen overlaid by the internal monologue of a director who is suffering from anxiety and depression; the monologue provides a detailed example of rumination and worry with its key themes of catastrophizing, overgeneralization, and self-criticism. To illustrate mental imagery, Ann Hackmann has used clips from the movie *Parenthood* to illustrate the way that mental imagery can encapsulate personal meanings such as people's worst case scenarios. Filming from the perspective of one person's inner perceptions is a technique that is used in many other films such as those of Alfred Hitchcock and David Lynch, and it can be used to illustrate how one individual's images can be mistaken for the objective narrative "truth" usually provided in film (see also Chapter 9, p. 186). This occurs in *A Beautiful Mind*, where the viewer is encouraged to see the protagonist's hallucinations as reality. In many of Lynch's movies there is little objective "truth" within the diverse fantasies that are portrayed. These themes can provide illustrations of metacognition, described in more detail in the next section.

Metacognition: the relationship with one's own cognitions and how to manage them

Metacognition has been defined in many ways. The simplest definition is *thinking about thinking*. More specifically, it refers to the monitoring and regulation of cognition (including attention, memory, thoughts, impulses, and imagery) through automated procedures and declarative information about one's cognition. While there has been a steadily increasing body of empirical and theoretical work in this area for over 30 years, its important implications for clinical populations are more recent, particularly owing to the work of Adrian Wells. There are two caveats that should probably precede a section on metacognition, and they both involve the way that the term is defined and delineated. First, whenever cognition is described, either in an empirical sense, or by our clients, there is often a simultaneous, implicit notion of metacognition. How else can we talk about our cognitions except through monitoring them and identifying them in the first place? Clients often report that they are "losing control of their mind" as their reason for coming to therapy. This implies that there is something in the mind, presumably a stream of cognitions, to be controlled in some way and that they are no longer able to do this. An implication of this first caveat is that the earlier sections of this chapter are likely to have features of metacognition too. This is because, as humans who can introspect, and *need* to introspect just to be able to translate their perceptions into words, we inevitably involve some form of metacognition in accounts of pure cognition. The second caveat is that, in trying to explain the regulation of cognition, the field of metacognition covers similar ground to other approaches such as certain cognitive models (e.g. OCD, Salkovskis, 1985), mindfulness-based cognitive therapy (MBCT), acceptance and commitment therapy (ACT), and the social mentalities approaches within CBT. The overlaps and dividing lines between these various accounts of how thoughts are monitored and regulated are not clearly described. Therefore, for the sake of parsimony, it will be assumed that as far as metaphors are concerned, they refer to much the same thing. Moreover it will become apparent that, with some exceptions, the metaphors tend to be shared across these areas. This is encouraging, as it suggests that each of these approaches is converging on a similar style of managing inner experiences that is helpful for our clients.

To begin this section, we will provide a therapy dialogue of a client-generated metaphor. We hope to illustrate that while metacognition and its associated incarnations can appear complex and depend on a large knowledge base, the experience of metacognition is universal. We each have our own ways of explaining it. Therapists may be able to start from the client's own way of explaining their metacognition rather than feeling that they need to explain a set of difficult concepts. The term "thinking about thinking" is a start, but there is a richness of our client's experiences that we could miss unless we listen carefully and try to understand their mental world.

Therapist: So, you're telling me that your thinking has changed now. Can you tell me how it has changed?

Client: At that that time I could think logically, and now I can't seem to. The way to describe it to you is that there is a brick wall there *(gestures to indicate a wall in front of him)* and I am going at it like that *(gestures with arms to indicate heading towards the wall)*. Right?

Therapist: Right.

Client: Like a square thing going at it, bang it's trapped.

Therapist: Just heading towards it?

Client: Straight into it. Bang. And there's my thoughts. There's no way of getting out of your thoughts that way, no way that way, no way that way and no way that way *(indicates left, right, up and down)*.

Therapist: Right, so you come into it here, and it's a straight brick wall, and you can't seem to get out of it left or right, or up or down?

Client: That's what I mean. You're like a square thing going at it. So you're trapped every way.

Therapist: So where are the walls?

Client: Just here *(indicating the front)*.

Therapist: So, how come you can't go left or right?

Client: Because you are trapped inside this square thing, and you hit it like that. And all you can see is the blackness of walls beside of you. And that's what's happening to my thoughts. They are catching on something, and it could be the most trivial thing.

Therapist: So you have this way of thinking, whatever the topic?

Client: Yes, whether it's finances, relationships, dark thoughts. It's either full on or nothing.

Therapist: So the topic can vary enormously.

Client: Yeah, it can. The subject is not important. It's the way of thinking. It makes me wary that these thoughts will just go on and on, and I get more fixated.

Therapist: So you don't want to go on down one line of thought too far?

Client: Yes, I don't mind if they are all jumbled as long as they are light thoughts. But when they are heavy, they overpower me. That thought becomes my life.

Therapist: So it's like you take these heavy thoughts with you and you head towards this brick wall and you feel like you can't get out of it?

Client: Yeah, yeah.

Therapist: Ok, and what happens the rest of the time?

Client: The thoughts are still in my mind, but it's OK.

Therapist: You're not right up against the wall?

Client: That's right.

Therapist: You're not fixated?

Client: Right.

Therapist: So what is different about the thoughts now?

Client: I don't know. My general thoughts, it depends on the circumstances. I could be laying awake in bed all night, and all of a sudden…

Therapist: So, that feeling of the brick wall only comes on in certain circumstances?

Client: Yeah. Other times I can take my mind off it, like I said. I've been staying in bed late, so I've had a lot of time to think about it.

Therapist: So, it's more likely to come on when you are laying in bed? That's when?

Client: Yeah. The thoughts completely envelop me.

Therapist: And it's similar to the worry that we talked about before?

Client: Yes. It's frustrating.

Therapist: It's difficult for me to know about what makes this happen. It seems to overlap with a lot of what we have discussed. What could be helpful is if you could monitor when you are thinking in this way, noting when this is like "a block heading at a brick wall." You said it happens in certain situations, so could we plot it to see when it is happening and when it isn't. How does that sound?

Client: Yes, I'll do that.

Therapist: The idea is that we can try to work out what situations help you manage your thoughts like you want to, and in what situations they hit this brick wall. Then, we may be able to work out how you can have more times when they are manageable.

In this example, the therapist is not trying to impose his model of how the client's thoughts get "fixated." He is happy to use the client's vivid metaphorical description and use this template to help him monitor when this cognitive style occurs and when it does not. It is likely that the process of monitoring will provide the client with an awareness of the contexts and consequences of this thinking style so that he can make his own changes. If necessary, the therapist and client can go through the monitoring sheets more systematically to develop a more detailed functional analysis.

In addition to helping clients articulate their own metaphors for how they manage their thoughts, there are likely to be situations when the therapist can suggest a prepared metaphor to the client. Within the literature on metacognition, there appear to be metaphors for both unhelpful and helpful metacognitive strategies, and it is these that we will turn our attention to next.

Unhelpful metacognition: Control of thought as a problem

The idea that struggling with one's own mind is a problem has been evident within cognitive behavioural therapies for many years, but it has gained more importance recently. Paul Salkovskis gave thought suppression a major role within his model of obsessive-compulsive disorder as one form of safety behaviour (Salkovskis, 1985; see also Chapter 7, p. 131). For example, if a client believes that their thoughts are a sign that they are an evil person, they will try hard to push these thoughts out of their mind. They begin to believe that they must continue to suppress these thoughts in order to remain a good person and stave off their evil side. Every time they fail to keep these thoughts away, they increase their efforts, until much of their time is spent carrying out elaborate rituals directed at keeping these thoughts from awareness. Often it seems that the harder one tries to suppress a thought, the more it appears, and there is some evidence to support this "rebound" effect. Probably one of the earliest metaphors to illustrate the futility of thought suppression was provided by Daniel Wegner through the "white bear" effect (Wegner & Zanakos, 1994).

Try as hard as possible not to think of white bears. Whatever you do, if you get the thought of a white bear, get rid of it! When clients try this exercise, they often find that when they try not to think of white bears, the thought of a white bear comes to mind. This may happen because in order to try not to think of a thing, you have to think of that thing first and then remove it from your mind, so the instruction to remove a thought actually contains that thought. This makes the task impossible to do faultlessly. Therapists we know seem to have their own different versions of this exercise. The white bear to not think about may be sitting on the therapist's shoulder; by all means feel free to substitute your own coloured animal!

Within later CBT approaches the problematic nature of thought suppression has taken centre-stage, most notably within metacognitive therapy (Wells, 2000) and ACT. Indeed, ACT makes explicit use of metaphors and prioritizes their use over more intellectual methods of intervention. We will not repeat the ACT metaphors in detail here, as they are illustrated very clearly in other publications (e.g. Hayes & Smith, 2005, p. 24, 36, 37). We particularly like their examples of the tug of war with a monster (the solution is to drop the rope, not to continue pulling!), feeding the tiger (every time you suppress you feed the tiger with more red meat so it gets stronger every day), and quicksand (in reality struggling in quicksand increases the chances of sinking, whereas stopping the struggle and lying down raises the chances of getting out alive).

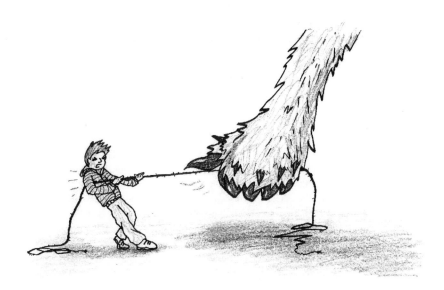

Unhelpful metacognition: Recurrent thinking as a problem

The flip side of thought suppression, it seems, is thought elaboration—the tendency to embellish thoughts with extreme personal meaning that is often negative or threatening. This way of thinking may come under different terms depending on its nature and content: rumination, worry, self-attacking. It contrasts with mindfulness, the awareness of the present moment in a none-valuative manner, which we will describe in the next section. It can be important to try to understand these experiences of our clients and develop shared metaphors for the process. Here is an example of how one therapist, Helen Morey, has approached it:

> I was trying to explain a metacognitive model of worry to a client the other day, and this was the image that sprung into my mind—a machine used to propel tennis balls. I talked about how my client seemed to be "constantly pelted by tennis balls of worry", and that she was trying as hard as possible to catch every one of them. In sessions where we dealt with each worry in turn, it had little effect, because another worry would be coming along in a few seconds. I suggested how the "tennis balls" that the person was getting pelted might be the same ones that most people had—the difference was that most people realized that most of the time you don't need to catch the ball, and that even if you can't manage to catch the ball right now, you could always pick it up again later. So, a metacognitive approach is about helping people to "stop catching the ball," and realizing that they don't need to.

Another example is the script metaphor. The idea is that that when we worry, we create a script in our lives of the worst series of events that might happen. By helping the client to explicitly generate a range of scripts, they begin to recognize the arbitrariness of each script and its loose relationship with reality, just like habitual worry. A similar metaphor of "bad news radio" is used within ACT. In this quote, the therapist Aidan Bucknall explains how he approaches the script metaphor:

> I asked my client to write several scripts for the next two hours of my life. In the first script I wanted the client to write a mundane script. This was talked through with the client: "I am gonna leave here. I am going to get in my car. My car will start. I will drive without incident to the gym. I will enter the gym without incident. I will do an hour's exercise. I'll feel a bit sweaty and so I will have a shower. Go back to my car. Drive home without incident. I will have my supper. I will sort out bits and pieces. I will read my mail and then watch a bit of telly and then go to bed". That would be the mundane version and you would need to think of a realist film maker, but it would be their film. The client would then be asked to write out several other version, one comedy, one horror, one action-adventure, etc, in 10 lines. The horror version was all blood and gore. The comedy version was the therapist slipping on a banana (see the movie *Clockwise* for some great examples of worst case thinking), and in the action-adventure script the therapist gets caught up in a situation similar to Jack Bauer in the series *24*. The client was perfectly capable of doing this. I then ask which one would be the

most likely to happen? The client typically replies: the mundane one. Which would anyone make into a film or which one would definitely not be made into a film? The client replies: the mundane one would not get made into a film. Which version would you automatically think of if you were living you own life? The client replied: the horror version straight away. So, the exercise helped to get the client to understand about the habitual tendency of entering that style of thinking.

Mindful awareness

There are a series of metaphors that seem to acknowledge both the helpful and the unhelpful styles of thinking within the same image—the mindfulness and the mindlessness, if you like. Here we provide three simple examples: the snowball, the cloud, and the train. There are more detailed examples within ACT (Hayes & Smith, 2005) and within metacognitive approaches, including an accessible, focused paper on "ten metacognitive techniques" by Adrian Wells (Wells, 2007).

We have each encountered clients who talk of how their mind seems to "snowball" when they are ruminating. One gets the sense that they start the process with some degree of control, but that the longer they engage in rumination, the more difficult it is to control, until their thoughts seem to feel unstoppable and out of control. In essence, this process is like rolling a snowball down from the top of a hill. The snowball is the initial thought, which might not have much emotional weight. However, it picks up snow as it goes down the hill, getting bigger and heavier and more upsetting, until there is an avalanche of distress. Yet in mindfulness, the snowball simply "skates off" the surface of our minds, as though the hill was made of ice, and we let it fall off the hill. We are not allowing it to build up snow as it moves along, but halting that tendency early on. Another analogy is to see your thoughts as clouds. So when you find yourself thinking about something this is as though you are riding on the cloud itself. Instead, try to step back down to the ground and observe that thought as a cloud in your mind, and then watch that cloud as it goes by. The train example is similar; instead of buying the ticket and getting on the "mind train," stay on the platform and watch your thoughts as they pass by.

Each of the above metaphors provides an image of how one can get "caught up" in one's thoughts, and a shift in perspective within that image that provides an alternative relationship with thoughts: the decentred, observing relationship that seems to encapsulate what we call mindfulness. In our experiences, clients vary in their readiness for exploring these exercises, and they are best accessed through discussions with clients of what they are already experiencing in their minds. Often these metaphors can then emerge from the client's description, much like the vignettes provided earlier. Nevertheless, these metaphors also provide an access point to experimenting with mindful awareness techniques in more directive approaches, and the emerging evidence is that they can be effective (Wells, 2007).

Facing problems

Sometimes mindfulness appears ambivalent about whether distressing experiences are to be attended to, or avoided. Is the process of decentring a way to create psychological distance from one's distress? Does the process of acceptance lead a person to be swamped by their inner turmoil? One way to conceptualize effective decentring is as a way to get a perspective on a problem such that it can be described and understood more effectively. One would gain little understanding of the problem through either allowing it to overwhelm one's awareness, or through suppressing it completely. This suggestion is quite subtle and may need a metaphor to explain.

Imagine that there is a fierce dragon lurking in the hills around your village, and has been attacking the townsfolk. You are the knight who has been charged with saving the village—quite a responsibility. What do you do? Would you charge the dragon's lair immediately with every ounce of energy you possess? Would you cower in the village church, praying to be saved but too afraid to even look at the dragon? Or something else? The second plan is clearly a non-starter. While the first plan has a greater likelihood of success, it has its risks and may backfire. Are you sure the dragon is in its lair? What weapons would be most effective? Will there be a trap? Presumably the solution is to gain more information before tearing in to the fiery cavern? From what perspective would you gain that information? Clearly not from the village church, and not by standing six inches away from the dragon's sharp teeth! You would gain information from going near enough to the dragon to observe it, and far enough to be safe. You never know, you might discover that it is just a little white rabbit, like in *Monty Python's The Holy Grail*! Even if you don't reappraise the dragon as something harmless, your observation of it from multiple perspectives will give you a better idea about how to defeat it than the first two options. So perhaps mindful awareness is really about providing people with the metacognitive skills to observe their own problems from different perspectives. And that's not just an example of using a metaphor to explain a theory, but a theory based on a metaphor!

Facing inner conflict

When our clients start to face their problems, they often realize that problems are of their own making: they are doing one thing that stops them from achieving another and they cannot find a way to manage these two goals. For example, they may set themselves perfectionist standards to try to overcome their feelings of failure but their pursuit of these standards leads them to fail in various aspects of their lives. We have noticed that this awareness of inner conflict is a productive step and it can be marked by clients' metaphors. Some very familiar examples include "being in two minds," "stuck between a rock and a hard place," and "a double-edged sword." This realization can open up discussion of the pros and cons of certain strategies and goals to help the client reach their own decisions. The metaphor can continue to be used and explored during this process. For example the client who talks about balancing priorities may describe that she is literally imagining how her priorities are weights on two sides of a set of scales. Therapy can provide the space for the client to explore these images and see how they unfold before their eyes, as they gradually become more aware of the nature of their difficulties and what is maintaining them.

Insight

As therapists, we hope that our clients will eventually change their unhelpful cognitions. There is evidence to suggest that this shift can happen at discrete points during therapy (Tang & DeRubeis, 1999). Yet change in cognition is clearly not unique to CBT and can be described in several alternative ways: a shift in perspective; an insight; a realization. Our clients have described it in several ways too: "it was like in those cartoons where a lightbulb has just come on"; "I felt this sudden change, like everything made sense—che-ching!" Some clients describe a moment when they hit "rock bottom" that seems to precede the changes they need to make. Having sunk to the bottom of the sea, they realize there is no further to go. Yet this feeling of a solid surface seems to provide some sense of safety. It seems to be a moment that they realize nothing can get any worse, yet from which they can begin to build themselves again.

Psychologists within this area of interest often refer to some apocryphal tales within the history of scientific discovery that describe moments of insight that arise after long periods of inner debate and consideration. Legend has it that that Archimedes grasped the theory of displacement within an instant as he sat in the bath and saw the water rise—"Eureka!" he exclaimed. Another historical account refers to the Austrian chemist Kekule who was working intensively to try to discover the molecular structure of benzene. According to the story, he dozed off in front of the fire and woke up suddenly recalling a dream in which six snakes were linked head to tail in a circle. At this point he realized that the structure must involve six carbon atoms linked in a ring. These two stories illustrate how insights can often come suddenly, and automatically, following a long period of deliberation. They may help clients and therapists alike to

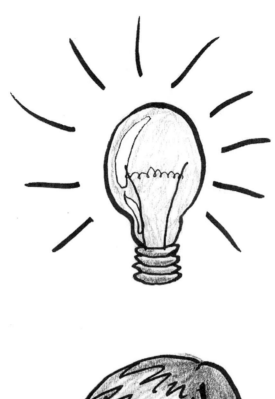

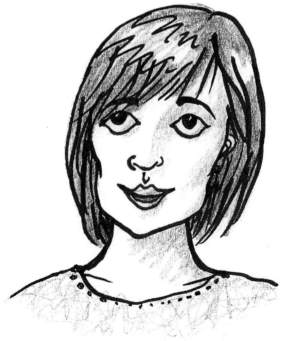

realize that the client's shift in perspective may not arise during the therapy session itself, yet the work carried out during therapy and for homework may be the important preparation that sets the stage for important changes in cognition. They make it clear that the change will come from within the client rather than from being imposed from outside. Finally, the parallels between great discoveries and personal discovery within therapy may be self-affirming for the client.

One more illustration of insight is worth mentioning. Superficially, one might regard it as trivial, as it comes from a popular cartoon. However, the level of understanding of life struggles and the mental processing involved are impressive and this is coupled by the ease with which a cartoon medium can provide vivid metaphorical images. *The Simpsons Movie* satirizes the cultural and literal notion of realization or "epiphany." As ever in this series of cartoons, Homer Simpson gets himself into serious trouble. This time he is responsible for an environmental disaster in his hometown of Springfield, yet he cannot understand peoples' extreme reaction to his little mistake. After he escapes the enraged townsfolk with the rest of the Simpsons, he is abandoned by his own family in the outreaches of Alaska. He wanders in the desolate snowy landscape, not able to decide whether or not to return home because he is so resentful at how everyone has treated him. We hear this internal dialogue reach a fragmented, staccato exchange of conflicting thoughts, until he eventually passes out in the snow. Fortunately, he is discovered by a kind and wise native Innuit woman who takes him into her home. She then encourages him to engage in a "throat singing" ritual to try to bring on his personal moment of epiphany. The audience is taken into Homer's inner dream world at this point, as we see him struggle with his problem against a backdrop of surreal grasping hands that try to tease the solution out of him. The hands pull at him until his own eyes are suspended in the air, looking at his own separated body parts. Eventually, after even the dream images seem to lose their patience, the shift in perspective occurs… "Oh I don't care about myself any more!… because other people are just as important as me… without them I am nothing… therefore to save myself I need to save them!"

The above sequence is rich in its exploration of personal problems and recovery, exploring themes of inner conflict, mindful states, self-reflection, and insight. Like in the more traditional accounts, change seems to come from within and from an experiential source, after a prolonged period of more verbal, conscious thinking. But clearly this account is not unique, and you and your client may have references within literature, film, television, and theater that reflect many of these processes. It may pay to watch some of your most loved films again, just to see where parallels can be made, both for your own thinking and for your clinical work.

Metaphorical systems: a client-generated example

To end this section, we would like to provide an example of the degree to which metaphor can permeate a cognitive behavioural approach to the most severe of psychological difficulties, and seem to aid in recovery. Mr Tolton had experienced a series of psychotic episodes until his eventual long-term recovery. He has documented this process in several articles (e.g., Tolton, 2005), each of which are rich in metaphorical description. He had received CBT through his care-coordinator, yet much of his recovery he puts down to his own use of poetry and metaphor. One insight that seemed to be important was the analogy between his memory of "psychotic information," which he termed the "rogue psychotic mindset" and other "mindsets," such as stores of knowledge about hobbies, family life and A-level subjects. He started to see this body of knowledge as a separate constellation of facts within his mind, and then took it upon himself to monitor his thoughts as they came into his awareness and make judgements as to whether they constituted psychotic or nonpsychotic information. He seemed able to "let go" of the psychotic thoughts and hang on to those that were more realistic. He reported using poems rich with metaphors as a way of engaging with this process:

Psychosis, disturbed thoughts, light, and hope
That thought was delusion,
I've nipped it in the bud.
I can recognize thought rubbish,
Split the factual from the dud.
I can separate the nonsense, from reality and fact,
From a muddled past existence, I am finding my way back.

Bedtime and the noise of thought
Lights out, sack time,
Time to rest your brain.
Switch off your thinking, rest the thought train.
Fidget-tappy-chatter, and the noise of flashback thought.
A loopy replayed daytime,
Then, by sleep, at last, I'm caught.

[Reproduced with the permission of Cambridge University Press]

Perhaps Mr Tolton's experience is too unique to set up expectations for our own clients. Perhaps the real mechanisms of his recovery were not those that he describes. Yet, his experience illustrates the potential personal importance of metaphor for establishing and maintaining mental health, and the extent to which it can be driven by the individual. Maybe our role as therapists is sometimes simply to sow the seed of insight in our clients' minds, water the growing sapling with care and consideration, and watch as it develops on its own.

Summary

Theoretical models of how the mind works can be hard to grasp. Yet metaphors provide a familiar bridge using everyday examples that are often vivid and memorable for clients. For example, "thinking about thinking," or metacognition, can be highly abstract without the use of metaphor. With the many colourful metaphors that are used in this field, it becomes a useful conceptual tool for clients to step out of unhelpful patterns of thinking. In particular, the therapist can be attentive to clients' spontaneous use of metaphors about their own thinking and help them to work through them and incorporate any change that is necessary. This can often lead to significant progress in therapy and set the groundwork for future collaboration.

Chapter 6

Depression

Introduction

Depression is a common problem and, for many, a debilitating one; it has been referred to as "the common cold of psychiatry." It adversely affects mood, enjoyment of activities, sleep, appetite, relationships, motivation, and confidence. Cognitive therapy began with a highly perceptive analysis of depression by Aaron Beck, who proposed that depressed people develop a set of cognitive structures of pervasive negative content centred upon the "triad" of the person's negative view of themselves, their current experiences and their future (Beck, Rush, Shaw, & Emery, 1979). This is linked to a pattern of negative attribution concerning events, referred to as internal, global and stable (*It's my fault, it will spoil everything and it will always be like this*).

Depression is often triggered by life events involving loss (e.g. bereavement, loss of role such as a job or in the family), but sometimes also happens without obvious cause. Sadness triggers off a pattern of negative thinking, which in turn further lowers mood, increasing the tendency towards negative thinking further, as a downward spiral. These factors lead to the development of self-maintaining cognitive processing biases, such as dichotomous thinking and selective attention, which act to maintain the problematic cognitions. Chronic and severe depression has been linked to the development of depressive "schemas" and "core beliefs"; such beliefs are believed to have the effect of modifying experience by altering and filtering it, resulting in "online" negative interpretations of current experience.

Cognitive therapy for depression typically involves the sharing of this understanding and formulating the client's problems. From early on in therapy, behavioural experiments emphasize the importance of behavioural activation and problem-solving. The client is supported in identifying potentially pleasant activities from which they have withdrawn or are avoiding with a view to re-engaging, thereby increasing the levels of positive reinforcement. Detailed discussion and behavioural experiments focusing on challenging negative beliefs identified as part of the shared understanding again focus on "finding out how the world really works" (see p. 38). A range of specific cognitive techniques are used to structure the process of belief change, including the use of continua, pie charts, and considering alternative less negative beliefs structured around strategies including the downward arrow and thought records (Beck, 1995).

More recently, research has extended to a more fine-grained analysis of factors such ruminative processing, mindfulness-based approaches, and behavioural activation. The cognitive behavioural treatment of depression has been shown to be effective for many individuals and offers some protection against relapse when compared to pharmacological treatment (e.g. Dobson et al., 2008). Nevertheless, many individuals still experience a chronic, recurrent pattern of depression despite treatment. Therefore, therapeutic strategies that can maximize and enhance the effectiveness of CBT are much needed.

This chapter explores the use of metaphor in the arena of depression. Beginning with a look at metaphorical descriptions of low mood, the chapter

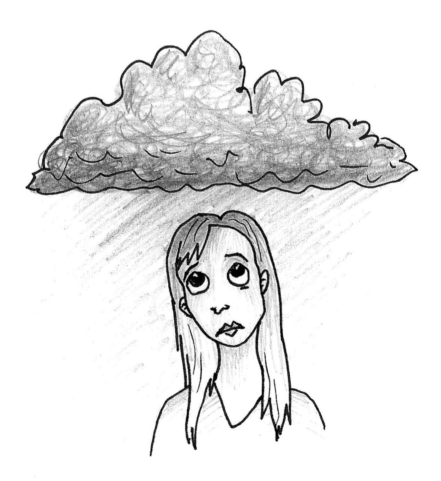

will then consider the use of metaphor in traditional components of Beckian cognitive therapy for depression, including thought identification, thought challenging, rules and beliefs, cognitive biases, the effects of isolation and withdrawal, and the persistence of schemata. Then the chapter will explore metaphor usage in more recent advances in different areas including behavioural activation, rumination, and the influence of self-criticism. Finally the chapter will consider the influence of past memories and take a brief look at mindfulness approaches in depression.

Our metaphorical language for low mood

Consider for a minute the myriad metaphorical ways people speak of depression. Perhaps most fundamentally, mood is oriented as if on a vertical axis—as up or down—as low or high. We experience a *dip* in mood, we can *sink* into depression, our mood can be on a *downward spiral,* we can be *down in the dumps* and we can hit *rock bottom.* Conversely, things may *look up,* we can experience a *lift,* we can be *on a high* or on *top form*—we might even, sometimes, reach *cloud nine.* However, we speak of mood not only by means of vertical position, but also by colour. Blue, sometimes. Black, also, of course. Winston Churchill famously described his episodes of depression as his *black dog,* symbolizing a sinister, ever present, and menacing companion. We speak of *dark* thoughts, a *dark* future, and of not being able to *see* our way forward.

Accurate listening to the client's own metaphorical language of depression can quickly reveal underlying cognitive structures that may need to be addressed. For example, the concept of *sinking* into depression is a metaphor of gravity—as if there exists an ever-present force seeking to pull us downward. A conceptualization along these lines is common, among people who are depressed, and is suggestive of themes including permanence, passivity, lack of control, and hopelessness. Cognitive therapy may wish to challenge many of these notions, and if the metaphor remains persistent and unhelpful, some creativity may be required to modify and restructure it. Sinking may need to be replaced by swimming, and the therapist might have to become a swimming coach.

In a similar vein, other clients speak of being *in the grip* of depression, or not being able to *shake off* their mood, or being *burdened by the heavy weight* of depression on their shoulders and thus unable to move. In each case, the metaphor can be inspected collaboratively with the client, often revealing the problematic cognitions such as restriction, loss of self-efficacy, and loss of hope. The following example illustrates how some gentle questioning on the

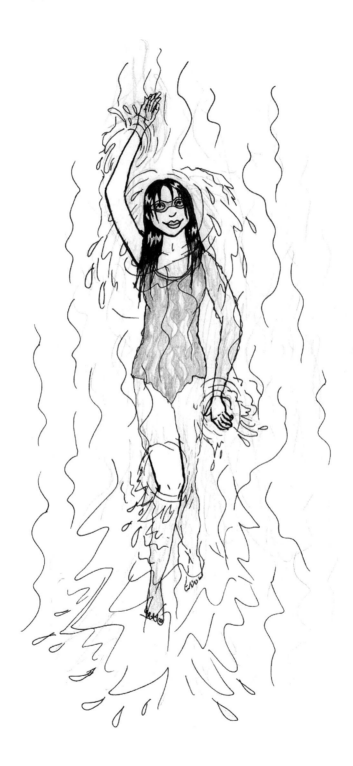

part of the therapist, and following the metaphorical language can elucidate the client's conceptualization of their problem:

Therapist: Can you describe a recent example when you were feeling low?

Client: Just all the time, really.

Therapist: You've been feeling low all the time, OK. That sounds pretty relentless.

Client: Yes. Doing anything is a struggle. Every little thing seems too much. I hate trying… I hate having to try all the time.

Therapist: I wonder if we can explore that? It sounds a bit like a battle—and one which you don't really want to be fighting in?

Client: Yes, exactly, I'm too tired to fight. I hate fighting. It's too much, too overwhelming. All I want to do is go back to bed, shut my eyes and not have to fight any more.

Therapist: Sure. And what happens when you do try and rest?

Client: I do spend a lot of time in bed. But then that isn't really a rest because I feel so crap for not doing anything with my life. I give myself a hard time. I lie awake and think about everything I should be doing, which drags me down even more. And I think, why should I have to fight, when other people seem to get up and live with no effort at all? That is not fair.

Therapist: OK, so it seems like you are really caught here—either you are battling your mood, which feels impossible and unfair, or else you are trying to rest but actually giving yourself a hard time—sort of battling with yourself I guess?

Client: Yes, you're right, I'm trapped.

This language in this short dialogue reveals that the client is construing their current existence as an unfair, unwinnable battle, against an overwhelming enemy, alone, ill-equipped, and with no possible exit. There are clearly many avenues to pursue here, and a variety of directions in which the therapist could usefully steer the discussion. However, this example highlights how simply following the metaphorical language has revealed some of the central cognitive themes, which are likely to be essential to tackle in the therapy.

Components of Beckian cognitive therapy

Identifying and challenging thoughts

An important aspect of traditional cognitive therapy involves identifying problematic thoughts and learning to challenge them with more realistic, helpful alternative perspectives. For many clients at the outset of therapy, the skill of identifying cognitions is an undeveloped one. Often clients get swept along by the emotional tide of their cognitions, without quite knowing what it is they

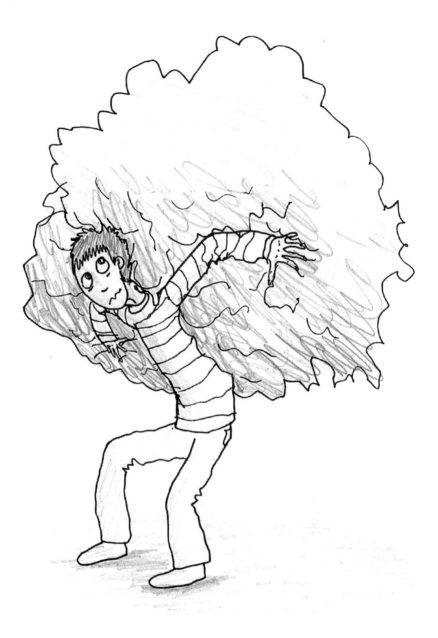

have been thinking. For such clients a useful metaphor to share is of the *mind as a train platform* (see also Chapter 5, p. 95). Thoughts are the trains that past through the station. Rather than rushing to jump aboard every train that arrives, the first task is to learn to be a good observer (train-spotter). Notice the trains as they come into the station, some of them going straight through, others pausing for a while and then moving off again out of the station. Notice the patterns of the trains too; the types that seem to come in regularly, as well as the less frequent ones. This simple metaphor can represent a significant shift of mind-set for many clients who may never have stood back and taken this observer's perspective on their own mental processes.

This metaphor emphasizes the "noticing" of thoughts, but in cognitive therapy we may also wish to think about and evaluate the validity of some of these thoughts. In an extension to the metaphor, this represents a change of role from train-spotter to rail inspector, complete with clipboard and official uniform. Now our job is to examine data on a particular train's performance, perhaps requesting surveys to be conducted or interviewing some passengers. Still, we don't behave in the old manner—rushing onto the first train we see. Our job is to weigh up the evidence and determine whether the train is acceptable, or is in need of updating, rescheduling, or complete cancellation. This metaphor can prove useful in assisting clients to evaluate problematic cognitions in a balanced and dispassionate way. It may be further enhanced by asking clients to visualize a busy local train station they know, and visualize themselves in role as a rail inspector, to consolidate the mind-set that is required. In short, clients can learn to engage with the content of thoughts when necessary while maintaining a degree of distance from the emotional power of the cognitive material.

Sometimes, clients present with almost the opposite problem, that of being numb or cut-off from their own thoughts and experiences. They may be mentally suppressing or avoiding their own thoughts, or are champions of distraction and thought substitution. They may exhibit overintellectualized discussion, or tangential dialogue, in order to protect themselves from entertaining the troublesome cognition or experience. The classic thought suppression experiment may be helpful here to highlight the ultimate futility of pushing away thoughts (see also Chapter 5, p. 92). The client is asked to try hard for one minute not to think about a white bear sitting on the therapist's shoulder, they are asked what happened, and what it tells them more generally about material we try to suppress. (Do please find a colour and a species you are comfortable with, though—one of the present authors finds that a purple hedgehog works well...)

Additionally, the experiential avoidance may be likened to wanting to avoid a bomb that might go off. While it is highly understandable to want to run a mile, this won't stop the bomb, and a better strategy is to decide to defuse the bomb. This emotive (and slightly alarmist) metaphor should be introduced carefully, but the hyperbolic message is often powerfully and memorably conveyed. As with the rail inspector metaphor earlier, this promotes approach rather than avoidance, and of a specific kind: careful, systematic, and professional. And taking the bomb metaphor one step further, perhaps it is only by carefully approaching in this way that one will discover there is actually no bomb at all, but only an innocent scrap of paper with the word "bomb" written on it.

Rules and underlying beliefs

There are a variety of ways that cognitive therapists describe the underlying, pervasive beliefs held by clients. Some therapists choose to distinguish between unconditional beliefs, known also as "core beliefs" on the one hand, and "dysfunctional assumptions" or "conditional beliefs" on the other (see also, Chapter 5, p. 85). A classic example of the former is *I am worthless*, and of the latter is *If I don't please other people I will be rejected*. Many of the client's thinking processes, interpretations of events, and behaviour patterns are seen to be built upon the architecture of these belief structures.

Terminology perhaps more user-friendly to clients is to refer to the underlying beliefs as "buttons which get pressed." Everyone has their buttons which get pressed—and so this is a normalizing, destigmatizing form of metaphorical language for the concept. It is also simple and visual; indeed some clients may benefit from drawing the buttons alongside the identified belief in order to lodge it in mind. Another term used by Fennell (1999) for core beliefs is of the "bottom line"—again this is easy to comprehend and captures the nature of the client's conceptual world whereby the ultimate meaning of adverse events often tends to boil down to their core belief.

Dysfunctional assumptions often map closely onto "rules for living." For example, an assumption that *People would look down on me if they knew the real me* might translate into an implicit rule *I must not share personal information with others*. In effect, a whole rule book may be operating. In some cases, the client may not be fully aware of the rules they are employing, but rather they have become habitual patterns of behaviour and thought. Rules often work in this way, fast becoming accepted, internalized, and unquestioned. The *traffic lights analogy* is a good one for understanding rule-governed behaviour—we tend not to question the rationale for a set of traffic lights to have been installed at a particular place, or question why it may be important for safety reasons or legal reasons to observe traffic lights—we simply stop when they turn red and go when they turn green.

If it is established that maladaptive rules are at work, it may be useful to consider with the client the idea of *rewriting the rulebook*. Once again, this is easily accessible language and is more closely tied to behavioural change than the abstract "modification of dysfunctional assumptions." Therapy may then take the work in different directions, but one common theme is of introducing flexibility into rules. The client has identified that they want stronger foundations for their life. Rigid rules often give the feeling of certainty, safety, and strength, but perhaps this is an illusion. Has the client ever wondered how it is possible to engineer buildings to withstand earthquakes? Is it by making them as rigid as possible? In part, actually, it is quite the opposite. Modern engineering, used in countries such as Japan, has developed a technology known as "base isolation," which effectively reduces the rigidity of the foundations of buildings. Instead, a flexible foundation is constructed, which is capable of absorbing and withstanding the massive horizontal forces of an earthquake that could otherwise cause fatal damage to the fabric of the building. This concept that flexibility can actually *increase* strength and resilience may be novel to many clients.

Another metaphor is to consider rules as *tools for a job*. Indeed, it is often found that rules held by clients have an adaptive origin, often in a different environment or in the childhood home. For example, an individual who grew up with an alcoholic and unpredictable mother may have developed a rule *I must be self-sufficient and never express emotion*, which may have been adaptive in this environment but becomes problematic later in life when they are unable to form close relationships with others. A tool for a job at one time may not be the right tool for a different job at a different time. The saying *Give a child a hammer and everything becomes a nail* captures the idea that it is easily to construe reality in terms of the tools with which we are familiar. However, much as we need a variety of tools for different tasks, we need different rules in order to adapt to different contexts and life stages.

A related metaphor is to consider assumptions as "personal contracts" of the form *If I do X (e.g. win other's approval) then Y will occur (e.g. I'll be happy)* (Beck et al., 1979). Such personal contracts may have been "drawn up" when the client was young, and as a result suffer from being overly severe or rigid. If this is established, the client might be asked whether, if he or she were running a company, they would allow a child draw up the contracts. The discussion could then acknowledge the understandable origins of the rule, but emphasize that the contract needs to be "renegotiated," or even abandoned.

Isolation and withdrawal

People who are depressed are often isolated or alone. In some cases this may be causal in their depressed mood—perhaps especially if a recent loss has occurred. However, often depressed individuals say they feel psychologically "cut off" even when other people are around. They feel as if there is a barrier between them and the rest of humanity. As time passes, the depressed person increasingly loses interest, motivation, energy, and drive to pursue activities and relationships, contact with others may lessen and before long there develops genuine isolation. The cognitive model then suggests that the isolated person has not only fallen into a habitual pattern of low activity, but is also subject to a barrage of negative thoughts, e.g. "No-one will want to speak to me anyway," "I'm no fun at the moment," "I've got nothing to talk about," "Other people haven't got time for me," "I'm just a burden," and so on. Therefore, cognitive factors conspire with the behavioural ones to maintain the isolation.

Metaphorically the essential themes here are being cut off by a barrier, losing human connection and being unable to escape this pattern. Dorothy Rowe (2003) captured this predicament succinctly—likening it to being *alone in a prison*. Sometimes clients will provide their own variants on this spontaneously. For example, they might describe feeling like they are in a pit, and not being able to clamber out. In other cases, the therapist may usefully characterize the situation metaphorically and ask the client whether this fits their feeling about how things are. Consider the following dialogue between therapist and client:

Client: I feel like I have absolutely no idea what I'm doing or where I am in my life.

Therapist: And how connected do you feel to others around you?

Client: Not at all. I have left them way behind. It's like I've been driving, blind, like not knowing where I am headed, and now I'm in some horrible tunnel that seems to have no end in sight.

Therapist: And this tunnel is a pretty dark place to be right now?

Client: It's hard to describe—like it's worse than dark. There's supposed to be a light at the end of the tunnel, isn't there, but I can't see any light—I don't even know which way to turn.

Therapist: That sounds a very difficult situation you're in. You don't know which way is forward.

Client: I don't know, I can't make any decisions.

Therapist: Well, I'm guessing that in the pitch dark it is hard to make decisions. But we have talked about one route forward, which is to make contact with your old friend Mike. And I suppose the other option is the "do nothing and wait" option. So there's a bit of a fork in that tunnel I suppose.

Client: Yep. But the "do nothing" one isn't really an option. That's just like a loop, which turns back on itself and gets me absolutely nowhere. I kinda know which tunnel I have to go down.

Therapist: Uh-huh.

Client: It's just—why can't I decide to do anything?

Therapist: Well, you did decide to get involved with therapy, and that's great because I'm able to come to this fork in the tunnel and help you shed some light on things.

Client: Yes, it is definitely clearer. I feel stupid for needing anyone to help me.

Therapist: Well, we all need help with things at times. What do you think your friend Mike would say?

Client: He's probably thinking, why's that total idiot stuck in the tunnel and refusing to come out! [laughing]

Therapist: OK, so he's on the outside, that's interesting, and presumably he's there waiting and watching because...?

Client: ...yeah, because he's a good mate I guess.

Therapist: So if we pictured that tunnel from outside in the full light of day, who else might be there?

Client: I dunno, my sis maybe, and maybe some other guys from the pub. I've never really thought there was people waiting outside the tunnel—I've only ever thought of it from the "dark" side, so to speak.

Therapist: That sounds important. So even though you can't see much light when you're deep in the tunnel, picturing it from the outside helps you see that there is light, and there are other people?

Client: Definitely.

Therapist: So what do you think you need to do?

Client: I guess I need to get back in the car, put the headlights on, and follow the "way out" signs.

In this extract of dialogue, the cognitive therapist tries to assist in subtly transforming the metaphor in ways that will advance the client's optimism and socialize them into a cognitive behavioural approach. The stuck, dark, trapped, indecisive themes of the metaphor are powerful components of the client's depressive predicament. The metaphor is molded into one in which there is conveyed a degree of choice, human connection, hope, and motivation.

Black and white thinking

A dichotomous, all-or-nothing, "black and white" thinking style is typical of depressed individuals, though not exclusive to the area of depression. It can be associated with perfectionism, inactivity, and a sense of worthlessness (e.g. *I can't do it perfectly so I won't do anything—I'm a failure*). Beck et al. (1979) characterized this form of thinking as primitive, where reality is chunked up in a rather childlike manner as "all good" and "all bad," rather than a more mature conceptualization of the world involving multiple dimensions and many shades of gray. The *continuum* is a widely used and useful intervention to help socialize and reorient the client to a quantitative, rather than qualitative conceptualization of their thoughts and beliefs (e.g. Padesky, 1994). In collaboration with the client, and to structure the dialogue, the therapist may frequently wish to draw a physical line, perhaps on paper or on a white board, to represent the dimension of interest. Thus, the continuum may be considered also as an implicit visual metaphor. Nothing so clearly depicts a spectrum of existence between two polar positions as a line drawn between two points. In so doing, the therapist assists the client in creating a cognitive bridge to a rich network of understanding of all things quantitative and continuous.

It can also be useful to appeal to certain aspects of life which clearly don't fit a black-and-white model, and it may be valuable to recruit this kind of "gray-scale thinking" in order for the client to think more adaptively and in less extreme manner about their own problems. For example, take the area of skill learning. Did the client ever learn to ride a bicycle? Did they ever fall off during learning? Why was this? Was this an abject failure, or was it a normal step in the learning process? Should a child who falls off a bike on their first go and says "I can't do this" have the bike taken away and be ridiculed? Or alternatively, what could be said to them? And what about the adequately competent cyclist who can cycle around town, but would never consider cycling competitively? Is this OK, or should everyone who gets on a bike aspire to be gold medallist at the next Olympic games? Indeed, would the world be a pleasanter, more desirable place if everyone were competing with everyone else at everything for the number one spot? Getting the client to think sharply about these issues can help convey the messages that shades of gray can be adequate, desirable and often essential.

Overgeneralization

Depressed people tend to overgeneralize the negative aspects of their experience and there is often a global bias to their negative interpretations. There are many ways to capture this metaphorically, often involving light and colour. Someone has turned the *electrical voltage* down in their home, so all the lights have gone dimmer than usual. Alternatively, they are *wearing dark glasses* so everything appears darker than it really is. If you know your client well, more graphic and provocative language may help lodge the concept in mind. The client is wearing their "shit-filters," perhaps—these are the glasses that only let the "shit" through!

Schemas

Negative self-beliefs are a hallmark of depressive thinking and low self-esteem, and their breadth and endurance in some individuals in the face of apparently

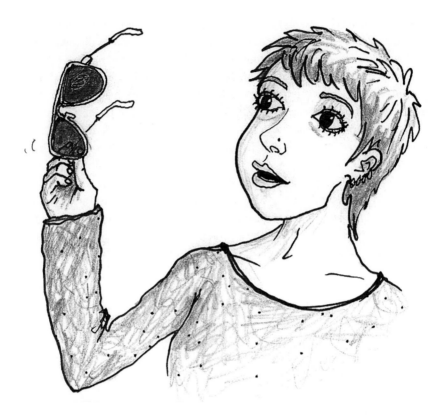

contradictory evidence is a fundamental cognitive puzzle that Beck et al. (1979) sought to address in the early years of cognitive therapy. At a therapeutic level, Christine Padesky (1990) introduced a powerful metaphor for the mainte- nance of negative schematic beliefs, conceptualizing schema as *self-prejudice.* This metaphor is introduced Socratically, first by asking the client if they know anyone who holds a prejudice, perhaps an acquaintance or colleague (a preju- dice which the client does not share) with a generalized belief that women can't drive, or that all builders are unreliable. Most often, clients will come up with an example, but if not then a prototypical or made-up example may be used, such as "women can't drive" or "all builders are crooks." The client is then asked to consider how the person would respond first to information support- ing the belief (a confirmatory example) and second, to information contra- dicting the belief (a disconfirmatory example). Typically, an asymmetry is brought out, whereby the person with the prejudice will notice and make much of the confirmatory example (e.g. *I told you so!*) but will ignore, dismiss, or discount the disconfirmatory example (e.g. *That's just the exception, yes, but that's only because X, Y, and Z*). The overall effect of these processes on the prejudicial belief is considered. Confirmatory evidence tends to strengthen the prejudice, but unconfirmed evidence is either not registered or dismissed, so the belief fails to weaken. Over time, the prejudice just strengthens and broadens. So, then, can the client see how this is relevant to their own beliefs? Is it possible that the client is following the same processes with their very own self-prejudice? Perhaps they are too easily seeing information in the environment as meaning they are worthless or unlovable, while readily dismissing information that contradicts their beliefs, e.g. information that they are likeable, worthwhile, or valuable. The final part of the prejudice metaphor seeks to ask how this problem might be resolved. Rather as the acquaintance with a prejudice needs some substantial evidence carefully pointing out to them, and is encouraged to pay proper attention and re-examine their beliefs, the client with a self-prejudice needs to devote more sustained time to spotting, recording, and processing the information, which supports a positive, alternative belief about themselves that may be more in tune with reality.

Yes buts...

Most cognitive therapists will have encountered the depressed client that seems to rebuff new ideas, suggestions, alternative perspectives with repeated "yes buts." For example, a suggestion of inviting a friend to have coffee to see whether they respond favourably is met with *yes but they would only agree to be polite*. It is almost as if the client has an internal drive to convince you, and themselves, that things *can't* change, that they really are incapable and worthless, or that behaving differently won't make any difference. They speak as if their depressed viewpoint is fundamentally correct, and any attempt to challenge it or offer alternative viewpoints needs to be squashed or batted away. One possible conceptualization of this process is of a schematic structure "fighting back" (Young, Klosko, & Weishaar, 2003).

The metaphor of an old belief or schematic structure *fighting for survival* may be a valuable one. Old dictatorial regimes, when seriously challenged by political newcomers, have rarely held up their hands and said "on reflection, you're absolutely right in your views, so how about we step aside and let you take over." More often there is powerful resistance, bloodshed, and dogged determination to cling on to power. However, before embarking on this way, or any related metaphorical road, there is some preparation work for the therapist to do. The premise first needs to be established that the old belief is a competing contender, rather than "the truth."

Therapist: So your boss seemed pleased with your work?
Client: Yes but I don't think he meant it.

Therapist: What makes you believe that?

Client: Because I don't stand out, like the others. I just do my job, and he knows I struggle sometimes and he's trying to make me feel ok about things.

Therapist: And what does that mean to you?

Client: That I'm useless.

Therapist: OK, so we're returning to the "useless" theme again? It seems like that particular voice is pretty strong inside your head right now.

Client: Definitely.

Therapist: OK, I'm glad you've recognized that, because it seems to me like at certain times that "useless" voice is louder or quieter—like you said that before you were depressed, it wasn't as strong?

Client: Yes, but at the moment it's just…everything feels that way.

Therapist: OK, now perhaps we could take a look at the process which happened a minute ago. When I mentioned that your boss was pleased with your work, what did you say?

Client: Um—I can't remember.

Therapist: I think your first words were "Yes but." You said "Yes but I don't think he meant it."

Client: Exactly. I always dismiss everything don't I?

Therapist: Well, it's really useful that you've noticed you sometimes do that. But would I be right that it's pretty automatic, like it's not really you but it's that "useless" belief bit that is doing the talking here? It seems like that bit wants to fight back when it is challenged?

Client: I think that is right, actually. It's so powerful.

Therapist: Powerful, right. That bit is a dominant voice in your head sometimes isn't it? But does that make it correct?

Client: Well it certainly feels that way. I feel useless. I know that I'm not completely useless, I suppose, but mostly I feel so bad I can't even think about it properly.

Therapist: So any other perspective on things often doesn't get a look in?

Client: Yes. I don't give any other views any airtime.

Therapist: That's really interesting. So this "useless" belief is *hogging all the airtime*, and is fighting away for attention, squashing any possible challenger before it can get established. Does that remind you of anything?

Client: Actually I was just thinking of the weeds in my garden. The few times I tried to plant any proper flowers they didn't last two minutes because of all the weeds taking over.

Therapist: Ah, right… OK. So they were the dominant species, even though they didn't represent what you wanted your garden to look like?

Client: Yes. And I suppose I should have taken more care of the flowers, and not allowed the weeds to take over.

Therapist: Well, I'm sure there will be plenty of time to sort out your garden in due course! But for you, perhaps now you can practice recognizing these *"weed thoughts,"* which will probably come up whenever you are looking at new evidence about yourself, like we just were.

Client: So if I think "Yes but" then I need to think "weed thought"!

Therapist: That would be excellent—you can practice spotting this process happening, and whenever you notice it, you can picture those weeds in your garden to remind you of what is going on.

Client: And try to nurture the other little thoughts, like the flowers.

Therapist: Great!

In this example, the therapist first established that the old belief was one perspective only (albeit a dominant one), without which the remainder would not work effectively. Then the therapist provides the seeds of a metaphor of the bullish, defensive old belief and for a moment it looks like the client is running with a "radio" analogy—an old belief "hogging the airtime." But interestingly, the client suddenly runs with a variant—the rampant weeds in the garden, taking over. The therapist makes a snap judgement that this is a good metaphorical vehicle to pursue, and it serves the purpose well. It is instantly meaningful to the client, and comes complete with a distinctive memorable image to link to the process of identifying "yes buts."

Other, simple metaphors can be useful to employ in therapy when discussing with a client the idea that a new perspective doesn't feel right at first. For example, it could be likened to the experience of wearing *brand new shoes* for the first time. Most people have had the experience of new shoes fitting in theory but "feeling odd" for a while. Here, it is useful to get across the idea that it is well worth sticking with a new perspective for a while—"road testing it," a little like you would with new shoes. Not rushing to judgement is a key principle in shifting attitudes and beliefs (for a related metaphor about "brushing teeth," see Chapter 4, p. 55).

Recent advances in depression

Behavioural activation

Activity scheduling was an important component of cognitive therapy for depression even in the earliest Beckian approaches (e.g. Beck et al., 1979). However, evidence from the past decade particularly highlights the importance of behavioural activation (BA) in treating depression. Indeed, the evidence from randomized controlled trials have shown that therapies that adopt behavioural activation as the principal intervention are at least if not more effective than standard cognitive therapy for depression (e.g. Dimidjian, Hollon, & Dobson, 2006). Therefore there is good reason to believe that some form of behavioural activation is a crucial part of CBT in the context of depression.

Typical hurdles to be encountered when pursuing a behavioural activation approach with depressed people include a lack of motivation to engage in the task, and a lack of enjoyment perceived when trying out an activity. These are highly understandable given the nature of depression, and so metaphor may be helpful in resetting the conceptual framework and expectations of the individual so that there is less danger of becoming disheartened or disengaging from the task. The metaphors of *kick starting the system* or *push starting the car* can be useful here. (Push-starting is the increasingly antiquated art of starting a car with a flat battery by getting a couple of friends to push the car to running speed and then engaging the clutch so the car's momentum drives the engine by reverse action and sparks it into life.) The important ideas to convey are that the initial approach is not the final approach (we won't have to push the car for ever), that it may not feel particularly natural or enjoyable at first (in fact may be aversive), but that there will be a follow-through effect such that the rest of the system will get going and normality will gradually return.

Relatedly, an *activity as medicine* metaphor may be used. With many antidepressant drugs, doctors will urge consistent compliance and will warn of that the real benefits may not be seen for some time after initial doses are taken. Activity may be similarly "prescribed" in this way (although the details of the activity schedule will be derived collaboratively). One strength of this metaphor is to suggest that if positive benefit or enjoyment from activity schedules is attained, this can be seen as a welcome bonus, but not necessarily to be expected. By construing activity as medicine, expectations are not raised that there will be an instant mood lift when activities are undertaken. Above all, it is important to avoid the trap of depressed individuals regarding their embryonic attempts at activity as more experiences of failure and thus giving up.

Rumination

Rumination is a prolonged or repetitive dwelling upon one or more cognitive themes. It is already metaphorical; "rumination" means "to chew over," as in cows "chewing the cud," and refers to going over and over particular ideas without regard to new input. It is a cognitive process found within a variety of disorders, but probably most studied in the context of depression (e.g. Nolen-Hoeksema, 1991; Watkins & Baracaia, 2002). Depressive rumination may be focussed upon a variety of concerns, such as one's past actions or behaviours (e.g. *Why did I say something so stupid?*) or one's current mood state (e.g. *I'm feeling so miserable*). The process of rumination is in many respects more notable than the specific content. It tends to be circular and repetitive, laden with unresolved and unanswerable questions, automatically triggered, and may, to the ruminator, carry an illusion of problem-solving but rarely results in any form of resolution or progress (see also Chapter 5, p. 94).

Metaphor can be helpful with rumination in a number of respects. Describing and labeling the process of rumination may be important, as people who ruminate often report only a partial awareness of the process when it occurs—as if it "creeps up on them." Clients may be given a basic definition of rumination and asked whether they recognize this process in themselves, and if so how they would describe it—perhaps what it might look like. Sometimes clients will offer a metaphorical description, and if not, some other people's descriptions can be shared; e.g. *thoughts tangled up like spaghetti*, like a *ferris wheel*

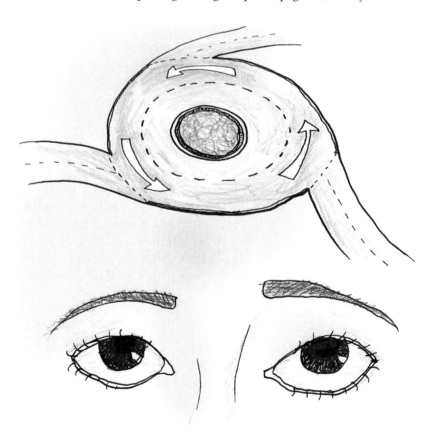

going round and round, racing out of control, and so on. Having a metaphorical description and image on which to hang the abstract concept of rumination is likely to be helpful in assisting clients to notice and to accurately label their mental experience. Sometimes the metaphors may then be extended creatively to move beyond mere description. For example, client and therapist could work together to slow down, step off and step back from the ferris wheel so that two feet are firmly on the ground. After all, when on a ferris wheel, it is hard to think about much else, but when both feet are firmly on the ground, one can choose to turn and look at much more in the world.

Another useful analogy is in tackling the usefulness of certain forms of questioning and berating of the self, which frequently occur in ruminative thinking. In particular, ruminators often ask themselves "Why" questions and hypothetical "What if..." questions. The client may be asked to consider for a minute a story (upon which there are numerous variants) of an *old woman who has tripped on a rug.* Two very different types of thinking could be employed at this point. One considers the needs of the old lady, and asks such questions as *What does she need?, How can I best help?, How might I rearrange the rug to prevent this occurring again?* It is about understanding but also problem-solving and moving things forward. A different form of thinking would be to repeatedly ask oneself *Why did this have to occur?, If only I had been there it might not have happened, What is wrong with me that I let this happen?, Why do things always go wrong when I'm around?.* Of course such thoughts are natural to entertain briefly, but if they persist and go round in circles then the system becomes "stuck" and little or no problem-solving occurs.

The client could be encouraged to consider what the important differences were between these forms of thinking. They could be asked which form of thinking is likely to be more productive and useful to the old lady. This analogy gets at the heart of a highly abstract notion—what is thinking for? A complete answer to this is thankfully unnecessary, but at least the client can be encouraged to consider their own ruminations, and whether this is equally stalled and unproductive. The metaphor of *conservation of mental energy* can be used also. The fact that the client is exercising so much mental energy ruminating suggests they are really keen to solve the problem of their current depression. But this kind of thinking is the wrong tool for the job, leaving them exhausted and fatigued, and no further forward. "Ruminating" their way out of their depression is not going to work, much as the old lady wasn't going to be helped by ruminating about the causes of her fall. That mental energy can be employed best in other directions, which can be discussed with the therapist.

Self-criticism

People with depression and low self-esteem are frequently self-critical. The language they will routinely use about themselves is harsh, evaluative, condemnatory, uncompassionate, sometimes surprisingly vicious and even bullying. In cognitive therapy, various techniques may be used to allow the individual to adopt a more balanced, compassionate perspective (Gilbert and Irons, 2004). One such technique is to separate the "bullying" and the "bullied" parts, to expose the inappropriateness of the harsh criticism. Suppose, for example, the client is criticizing themselves for having not passed a driving test (*I am such a loser, I couldn't even pass a simple stupid little test, I'm so crap*). The therapist might step into the shoes of the client and ask *If I made the mistakes you have done would you despise me for it?* And relatedly, *How do you think I would perform if somebody was standing over my shoulder criticizing and evaluating everything I did?* Another variation on this theme that can help is to ask the client to imagine a "gargoyle of depression" sitting on their shoulder (Otto, 2000). This gargoyle weighs down heavily and tries to blame the client

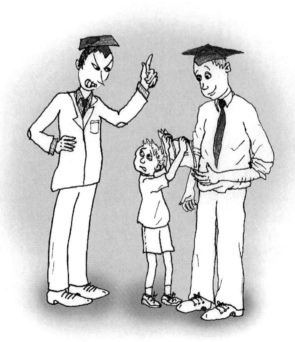

for that weight, hoping that they don't turn their attention to disposing of the gargoyle. This idea can be extended and elaborated, with the gargoyle whispering unfairly, in a relentless, harsh critical voice, which the client has to acquire the ability to recognize and label for what it is—the "depression gargoyle." Then a new, more compassionate voice can be used, modeled by the voice of the therapist.

Along similar lines, let's imagine a country where there are trialing two different *teacher training programmes*. In one programme they train up the teachers that if pupils are struggling or making mistakes they should be criticized, shouted at, bullied, and frequently called names like stupid, crap, and hopeless. In the other system they train the teachers to show warmth and encouragement to pupils, praising their strengths and supporting them when they are struggling with extra help and compassion. Which programme produces the more confident and happy pupils? Which system gets pupils to engage in their homework and develop their knowledge and grow as individuals? Which system is more likely to result in pupils being scared of learning? Which system should the government invest in? (See also Otto (2000) for a closely related story about two baseball coaches.)

Often this metaphor allows the client to realize the gross inappropriateness by which they are treating themselves and addressing themselves linguistically. The gentle humour invoked by this metaphor also facilitates processing and reappraisal of the entrenched self-critic. The next step for the client is to spot themselves falling into this trap and to develop a more compassionate and appropriate attitude towards themselves. For example, Lee (2005) has described a "perfect nurturer" imagery technique, which seeks to cultivate an imaginary compassionate figure capable of fulfilling the "soothing needs" of the individual. Through careful construction with the help of the therapist, and rehearsal, this image then becomes more readily available to directly counter the harsh self-critical voice that has previously been dominant for the individual.

Influence of past memories

Traditional cognitive therapy approaches to depression involved identification and modification of idiosyncratic belief systems, typically codified as propositional statements, varying in breadth and scope, relating to the self, the world, and the future. However, more recently there has been some interest also in the systematic influence of past episodic memories in depressed people on cognitive processing (Wheatley, Brewin, Patel, Hackmann et al, 2007; Brewin, Reynolds, & Tata, 1999). It has been shown that depressed individuals are prone to experience intrusive emotional memories, often involving themes of loss and interpersonal crisis. There has been some exploration of imagery rescripting techniques that facilitate processing of past "hotspots" of trouble-some memory, in order to remedy cognitive processing in the present (Wheatley et al., 2007). Ann Hackmann has described these memories as *"ghosts from the past,"* a helpful metaphorical turn of phrase when discussing the process with clients. Indeed, this metaphor succinctly captures the idea that past memories may continue to exert an intrusive influence beyond their apparent life span. Additionally, it may be useful to characterize this continu-ing influence as the *memory talking*. Again this captures the idea of the memory continuing to operate when logic would suggest it had been put away, processed, or finished with.

Much of the conceptualization of the cognitive processes at work here derives from theories of emotional processing, which take centre-stage in the treat-ment of conditions such as posttraumatic stress disorder (Ehlers & Clark, 2000) as well as borderline personality disorder (Young et al., 2003; Weertman & Arntz, 2007). The facilitation of emotional processing might be thought of as "finding a place for the memory," or perhaps "laying the ghost." We also discuss metaphors for emotional memories in Chapter 5 (p. 85) and Chapter 7 (p. 151).

Mindfulness approaches

Jon Kabat-Zinn (1994) quotes the caption on a poster of an elderly yogi, Swami Satchitananda, shown riding a surfboard off a Hawaiian beach. It read "You can't stop the waves, but you can learn to surf." This rather wonderful quotation distils something of the essence of a mindfulness approach, which has been an important area of growth over recent years in the treatment of recurrent depression. These developments have been dubbed the "third wave" therapy approaches (see also Chapter 5, p. 95). In particular, an approach called mindfulness-based cognitive therapy (MBCT; Segal, Williams, & Teasdale, 2002) is a program developed to help protect individuals who have experienced multiple episodes of depression from future relapse. People who have previously experienced depression appear to exhibit a vulnerability such that that even a slight dip in mood may trigger a downward spiral of mood and negative cognition. This may be conceptualized as *grooves in a track*. Each time the connection between negative thoughts and negative moods is made, the groove deepens. Alternatively, these vulnerabilities may be thought of as *fault lines*, such that even when the depression is in remission, it takes less of a knock for the cracks in the ground to reappear and thus to slip through.

Another widely used metaphor is that of *floundering in quicksand*. This is a useful one because it carries an implication about the individual's probable response, and the danger of this response. Quicksand is a mixture of fine sand and water, and can behave in a treacherous manner by appearing solid but going liquid when weight is exerted on it. The person who instinctively fights back is more likely to get dragged down further due to added movement and pressure on the quicksand. The cool individual who has previously read their survival manual will know they should keep as still as possible to prevent worsening the predicament. In mindfulness approaches to depression, the theory is that people are likewise fighting too hard to free themselves from the grip of their low mood. They are engaging excessively with the content of the low mood in order to try and "solve" the problem of their depression, to work out why things are bad. Inadvertently, this backfires, as it ends up deepening the spiral of negative cognition and mood. Individuals need to adopt a different set of tools to tackle the issues they face, rather than the engaging, fighting, and ruminating ones. They need to know it is OK to try and stop "solving" the problem of their depression.

Mindfulness philosophy is sophisticated and cannot be described in full here. Most practitioners recommend that the techniques require practice to develop, and a nonjudgemental, accepting stance be adopted to the process of learning itself. Some of the key themes to convey the spirit of mindfulness are of nonjudgementality, acceptance, observation, being in the present moment, not striving or resisting, being acutely attentive but distanced and being able to let go. It is said to be about "being" rather than "doing." Observing *clouds crossing the sky* captures something of this stance metaphorically. Clouds come and go, they are just there. We can easily see the futility of labeling clouds as good or bad, of trying to resist them, of pulling them towards us or pushing them away. We can just be in the moment, noticing them come and go, for what they are. We don't have to evaluate them or make any decisions about them. We can become fully absorbed in the experience of observing the clouds, and yet we are on the ground looking up and so we are separate from them. Interested readers can consult a number of excellent texts on mindfulness and cognitive therapy (Segal et al., 2002; Williams, Teasdale, Segal, & Kabat-Zinn, 2007).

Summary

This chapter has explored the use of metaphor in the arena of depression. We began with a recognition that everyone has numerous implicit metaphorical structures in their conceptualization of mood and well-being, which emerge in our everyday language. Hence we are low, we are blue, we are sinking, or struggling. Attending to the client's metaphorical language offers a valuable insight into their problematic cognitive structures, and a possible opportunity for constructing new, more adaptive "cognitive bridges." Metaphor was also seen to assist and bring to life some of the essential traditional components of CBT for depression, as well as some of the more recent and promising avenues for intervention including ruminative processing, imagery rescripting, compassion, and mindfulness.

Chapter 7

Anxiety disorders

Introduction

The central cognitive theme in anxiety disorders is the exaggerated appraisal of threat; that is, the client who suffers from an anxiety disorder mistakenly believes that what is happening to them is more dangerous than it really is. A commonly used metaphor that reflects the role of this theme in anxiety disorders is that of a "false alarm," where the person responds to an ambiguous situation as if it were extremely dangerous. To the anxious client, the false alarm progresses to become an emergency.

Increased levels of threat appraisal also occur in normal increases in anxiety, but the appraisal of threat is commonly mild or moderate and rapidly subsides with the passage of time. By definition, the experience of normal anxiety does not interfere significantly with the person's life, and the experience of threat is broadly consistent with the actual level of danger, with the appropriate mobilization of coping resources. Clearly the normal/abnormal distinction is dimensional rather than categorical, and indeed a key component of treatment is "normalization."

To understand "abnormal" anxiety (anxiety disorders), one must consider firstly why, for some people, anxiety ceases to be a useful alerting mechanism and becomes severely distressing and disabling. Secondly, we need to address the question of why people suffering from anxiety fail to benefit from the repeated experience of surviving anxiety-provoking situations unharmed. In behavioural terms, the principal metaphor used to account for these issues has been learning theory; this has been framed as the acquisition of conditioned emotional response through associative learning, and the subsequent failure of phobic reactions to extinguish in the face of unreinforced presentations of the conditioned stimulus (Eysenck, 1979). For the cognitive theorist, it revolves around the way sufferers misinterpret stimuli and situations as more dangerous than they really are, and the consequent overperception of threat (Beck, Emery, & Greenberg, 1985; Salkovskis, 1996). This chapter will first review the central themes of threat appraisal and the alternative explanation, before looking at some valuable metaphors that can be applied across anxiety disorders, and within specific disorders.

Threat appraisal and the alternative explanation

Why is the person's anxiety particularly severe?

The *severity* of anxiety an individual experiences can be understood in terms of the interaction between not only the perceived probability that something bad would happen but also how bad it would be if it were to happen. Most clients will be familiar with the concept of elevated probability of threat but the role of "awfulness" is often less obvious to them. For example, the agoraphobic client who fears fainting often doesn't just feel it is likely that they will pass out, but it is also implicit that once they have passed out people will ignore them, leave them lying there or that dozens of people will gather round and make fun of them, and so on. The idea that they might faint tends to come to the fore when the client is in a feared situation, while the "awfulness" component tends to be implicit until specifically examined in therapy. A further factor is the client's perceived ability to cope if the threat were to materialize. Such coping can be not only from the person's own resources, but also from external "rescue factors," things which might have the effect of making coping with the negative outcome easier, or even remove it altogether. The subjective level of threat can be expressed schematically, using a mathematical "formula" as a metaphor:

$$\frac{\text{perceived probability of threat} \times \text{perceived cost/awfulness of danger}}{\text{perceived ability to cope with danger} + \text{perceived "rescue factors"}}$$

Having identified both the perceived probability in a given situation and the linked "awfulness," helping the client understand that can be done by illustrating how even positive things can make you feel more anxious. For example, one of the authors describes having a mild fear of flying, which worsened fifteen years ago. The client is told that the reason it worsened is to do with his perception of how awful it would be if he was involved in a plane crash. After some discussion it is identified that what happened fifteen years previously was that his daughter was born. Before that event, the idea of being involved in a plane crash meant, of course, fear, suffering, and death but now had the added component of not seeing his daughter grow up, her not having her father there to look after her, and so on. In this way he illustrated not only the concept of awfulness, but also that positive factors can increase anxiety; and obviously negative factors can do something similar.

A range of stressful situations can be used to help the client understand how these factors work and interact with each other; in the course of such discussions, the therapist repeatedly seeks to make the comparison with the particular pattern of anxious appraisal the client is experiencing. An example is the *trainee air-traffic controller*. The client is asked to imagine that they are working on a flight landing simulator. You see two planes on your screen moving a bit too close and are quite concerned. You judge that the likelihood of a crash is very low, but you don't want to mess this up, because you want to pass this stage of your training. However, compare this to your first real assignment, the likelihood of failing to prevent a crash would be the same, still low, but the awfulness would be vastly increased, because it would not be just your training programme at stake but the lives of hundreds of people. Therefore, the perceived threat would be higher. If the two planes were actually headed straight for one another, the likelihood would be increased, therefore, yet more perceived threat. However, if you knew that at any time, you could calmly speak to the pilots and redirect their course, and they would invariably do exactly as you request, then your perceived coping resources are increased, and hence your perceived threat would be lowered. If you knew that another highly experienced controller was dealing with one of the planes, this would further reduce the sense of threat.

Why does anxiety persist when the feared consequences don't occur?

In the normal course of events, repeatedly encountering situations perceived as threatening will, in the absence of the anticipated harm occurring, lead to a progressive reduction of anxiety; in behavioural terms this is known as "habituation" or "extinction." So how does cognitive theory account for the evident failure of clients to learn from what appear to be repeated experiences of bad things not happening (Seligman, 1988)? On the face of it, this observation represents a serious challenge for cognitive theory (and associated therapy) given the clear normalizing philosophy. If the logic of the cognitive account of anxiety disorders is as straightforward and clear as is supposed, why does the logic of disconfirmation in the face of contrary evidence not hold equally? In other words, why does the panic client who believes that she will faint still believe this after approximately 2,000 attacks where fainting did not occur? Why does the obsessional person who fears contamination not lose their fear in the face of their continuing robust good health?

The cognitive theory provides a clear account of this (Salkovskis, 1988, 1996; Clark 1999), and the practicalities in individuals suffering from anxiety can readily be identified and clarified if the anxious client is asked the appropriate questions. The panic client who is asked why they did not die in the supermarket will tell you they would undoubtedly have done so had they not left *just in time,* or sat down and taken the strain off their heart and so on. The socially anxious person who is not laughed at when meeting people will tell you that this can be explained by the fact that they remained silent while others in the group had a conversation. The obsessional client will tell you that they did not act impulsively because the violent thought was resisted and then neutralized by a "good" thought.

Such safety-seeking behaviour is not necessarily pathological. "Avoidance" responses are characteristic of some normal anxiety. The behaviour of anyone who believes himself or herself to be in danger will usually focus on anything that he or she believes may reduce the danger or otherwise make them safe. Safety-seeking behaviours are a highly adaptive type of response where real threat is concerned. People leave a burning building as quickly as they possibly can. However, if the perception of danger is in the first place based on an unnoticed misinterpretation, then the safety-seeking behaviour can prevent the anxious person from discovering that their fears are groundless. After an episode that should have established that the feared consequence did not happen, the person who is engaged in active safety behaviours may believe that they had a lucky escape because they did things that prevented the feared catastrophe from coming about. From this perspective, the panic client who has had 2,000 attacks where they did not faint perceives themselves as having had more than 2,000 attacks where they were on the verge of fainting and were only just able to prevent it from happening. Safety-seeking behaviours can be global behaviours such as avoidance and escape, or more subtle forms of avoidance occurring within a situation which the person feels prevented a danger from materializing.

Cognitive theory of the maintenance of anxiety disorders

In terms of the maintenance of anxiety disorders, the cognitive-behavioural model incorporates the role of threat appraisals and safety-seeking behaviours as particularly important aspects of a general theoretical account of the maintaining factors as illustrated in Figure 7.1.

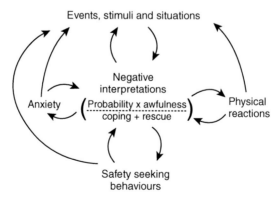

Fig. 7.1 General cognitive-behavioural model for maintenance of anxiety disorders.

An event or situation, for example a social interaction in a social phobic client, palpitations in a panic client or an intrusive thought in an obsessional client, are misinterpreted in a particularly negative way, as being more dangerous than they really are. These negative interpretations drive a range of reactions such as mood changes (e.g. feeling acutely anxious), physiological changes (e.g. heart racing), and cognitive changes (e.g. selective attention). In addition, they *motivate* safety-seeking behaviours as described above.

In people who suffer from anxiety disorders these reactions have two effects. First, they can maintain the negative meanings that the client attaches to them. For example the panic client, who sits down when they notice their heart pounding, then thinks that sitting down stopped them from having a heart attack; the social phobic who wore concealing clothing, so that sweating would not be noticed, believes that their clothes were the only reason that other people didn't comment on their sweating. Likewise, an obsessional client might believe that their loved ones didn't die of a fatal infection because they washed their hands sufficiently to get rid of it.

The reactions to threat may have a further unwanted effect; in some circumstances they may also increase the perception of experiences that were the initial source of misinterpretation and therefore anxiety. This type of effect is particularly obvious in obsessive-compulsive disorder. By definition, obsessional clients experience intrusive thoughts which they "attempt to suppress or neutralize by some other thought or action" (DSM IV, American Psychiatric Association, 1994). The deliberate attempt to suppress naturally occurring intrusive thoughts demonstrably increases the occurrence of these thoughts (Salkovskis and Campbell, 1994; Trinder and Salkovskis, 1994; see also Chapters 5, p. 92 and Chapter 6, p. 109). If the reader were to attempt to exclude thoughts of giraffes from the mind at this moment, it is almost inevitable that such thoughts or images would occur more frequently throughout the time that the active attempts of suppression were taking place. This is almost certainly due, in at least part, to the fact that the person is paying attention to the idea of giraffes. It is also self evident from the exercise itself why the "unwanted" thoughts are occurring. However, in the case of an obsessional client who is experiencing blasphemous or other types of unwanted thoughts, it is considerably less obvious. Such clients often think that the unwanted thoughts are occurring at an alarmingly high frequency when he or she tries not to think them; it therefore follows that thoughts would occur yet more frequently and in a more uncontrolled way if he or she were to cease attempts at suppression.

It is not only in obsessional problems that reactions to threat appraisal increase the symptoms that have a focus of anxiety. In clients anxious about their health it is not uncommon for lumps to be palpated or rubbed until they are painful and swell more, for medical tests to be sought with such determination that enough tests are conducted to give several false positive results, and so on. Counterproductive strategies of this type can be described and explained using simple metaphors such as "digging to get out of a hole" (see Chapter 4, p. 61).

From theory to therapy: constructing a bridge between understanding and application

As described in Chapter 3, a key element of cognitive-behavioural therapy is to help the client to understand "how their world really works." It helps, of course, if the therapist knows how the client's internal and external world really works too; if, in addition, they have a good grasp of empirically grounded theory of emotional problems, they then have a fighting chance of being able to work with the client to help them to begin the process of understanding and dealing more effectively with their problems. Part of that process is helping the person understand the factors involved in the persistence of their anxiety and to use this understanding to try different ways of reacting. The way the "shared understanding" (derived from the specifics of the cognitive model shown in Figure 7.1) is presented to the client is as a "vicious flower"; that is, as a series of interlocking vicious circles which converge on the negative appraisal. This itself can be regarded as a metaphor (see later).

Across the anxiety disorders a number of metaphors allow the client to make sense of the key maintaining factors in their anxiety and how these link to cognitive behavioural theory. Many of these will apply regardless of diagnostic group and are described next, followed by disorder-specific metaphors.

Factors occurring across anxiety disorders

Selective attention: "looking for trouble"

Clients will often demonstrate a heightened sensitivity to the detection and recognition of experiences in either themselves or their environment that they believe might be dangerous to them. Attention tends to be drawn quickly and selectively to such cues. Such an attentional skill has clear adaptive value when used, for example, to spot predators when one is away from safe places, or, perhaps of more modern relevance, cars when crossing a busy road. Many clients find such evolutionary arguments to be a helpful metaphor explaining such reactions. In an anxiety disorder, where threat is overestimated, this useful system can become a factor maintaining or increasing an already elevated perception of danger. In a panic client, for example, innocuous experiences, such as the natural fluctuations in heart rhythm, may be monitored closely, making variations (such as heart going faster, skipped beats) more obvious, and these being registered by the person as further "potential threat" signals. Note also that, as the person remains focussed on a potential source of threat, they become more skilled at detecting variations and nuances in that domain. Both of these factors makes the feared outcomes seem more likely in the client's mind, further raising anxiety levels and in turn perpetuating this tendency to attend in this selective way.

The metaphor related buzz-phrase here is *"looking for trouble."* Most clients, when asked what you find if you look for trouble will respond by saying "trouble," and that looking for it means that they are more likely to find it. Specific concrete examples may be useful to illustrate how the attentional system

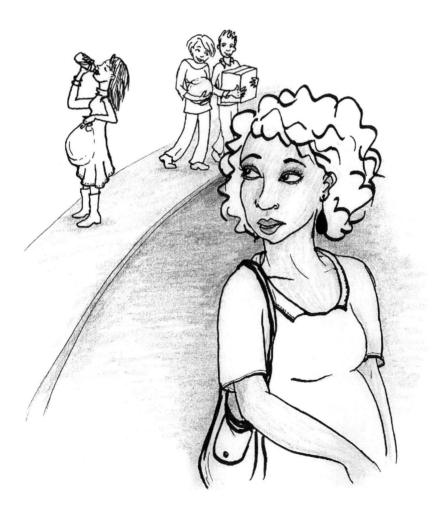

selectively brings personally significant perceptions to mind without there necessarily being any "real" change in the world. For example, women who have been pregnant may recognize (or remember) that they tend to notice other pregnant women and/or young babies when they walk down the high street. Similarly a new dad may selectively begin to notice other fathers with kids, whereas before he paid them little attention. The person who has recently *made a new purchase*, e.g. a new car, pram, jumper, or special pair of boots, can be asked if they then noticed more similar examples in their every-day environment. Another example familiar to many people is when learning or *coming across a new word*. Suddenly, it seems as if everyone is using this word at once! Every third sentence someone seems to use the word. The core elements of these selective attention metaphors are that the attentional system can become "primed" to spot certain things that have become personally relevant, that this process can proceed automatically and out of awareness, and that there may be a resultant illusory feeling (e.g. that the world is full of blue baby buggies).

Note also that deliberate efforts to make oneself safe can also have the same effect. However, although the person might know that they are scanning to be safe, they are not aware of the impact of this effort in terms of highlighting danger cues; the therapist can use metaphors, analogies, and related examples to help them see how this might work. When there is a bomb warning in the area you are in and you look for suspicious items or people, you find that there are lots (e.g. illegally parked cars, worried looking people carrying large rucksacks).

Anxious attention can also impact in another way; it can make you better at identifying things that have always been there but have usually gone unno-ticed. It has been shown that panic clients not only notice their heart beating more than others, but they make fewer errors in heart rate estimation (that is, they are more accurate at telling what is happening to their heart) (Ehlers and Breuer, 1992). Similar effects are almost certainly present in other disorders, and it is helpful to offer an account of these. A useful metaphor to help people understand the way this works is to ask them if they have noticed any birds as they went about their daily business. Sparrows? Starlings? Pigeons? Did they notice the different plumage of males and females? What would an expert bird watcher (who spends much of their time watching out for different birds) say if they were asked the same question? Why? A more directly relevant example for panic or health anxious clients would be comparing a psychotherapist lis-tening to the clients' heart beat with a cardiologist doing the same thing. What would a cardiologist hear? Why would that be different from the psychothera-pist? The therapeutic aim is help the client to reach the conclusion that they have become particularly expert in things related to the issues that they fear in the same way as a cardiologist is expert in heart sounds. For social phobics, the example of a "body language" specialist may be helpful.

The role of personal relevance (especially threat) in the overrecognition of threat can be understood by considering the role of two different radar operators; weather radar and air defence. For the weather radar operator, not noticing a blip on their screen means, at worst, that London gets an unexpected shower of rain. By contrast, if the air defence radar operator misses a blip, then London is destroyed by a nuclear bomb. The client is asked: Why is the second radar operator so much more sensitive to small events on his radar screen? What is the effect of this on how they react to what is going on in their radar screen? It means, of course, that the person notices more "false alarms"; the client is asked if it is possible that the same thing is going on in their case? How do you react to your "radar screen" when you are worried? Can you think of examples of that?

Perceptual narrowing: "zooming in"

A common consequence of anxiety is a shift in attentional range; either a narrowing (most common) or sometimes broadening of attentional focus. This can be likened to a spotlight in the dark, picking out particular threatening things (e.g. enemy bomber in wartime). Initially the beam may be diffuse while the person is scanning for threat, zooming in and focussing once a particular source of threat is identified. This is helpful when people seek to understand the "sharpening" of their attention when threat has occurred. It can also be compared to the "gun barrel effect" during armed robberies; "I don't know what he looked like, I just saw the hole in the end of the gun barrel." This helps explain why an anxious person becomes preoccupied with one aspect of a situation where they are feeling panicky to the complete exclusion of other details.

Safety-seeking behaviours: "the solution has become the problem"

Safety-seeking behaviours as described above are invariably voluntary responses, meaning that the client chooses to exhibit them. It therefore follows that they can choose not to exhibit them, and if framed in the right way, the result will be that the threat appraisal is reduced or eliminated. However, to choose *not* to use safety-seeking behaviours, or to carry out behavioural experiments testing out the reality of their feared disaster, requires both understanding and determination. The integration of metaphors into this process can be particularly helpful. These are described below in terms of different types of safety-seeking behaviours.

Avoidance: "keeping your head in the sand"

Behavioural avoidance is the narrowing of the behavioural canvas, such that feared stimuli are reduced or eliminated. Cognitive avoidance is the attempted reduction of certain mental material, often by suppression or distraction. Clients with anxiety problems are often insightful about some of their avoidance, and sometimes enter therapy with the popular metaphor of knowing that they need to *face their fears*. In our opinion, this metaphor should be treated with some caution, because for some it may carry an implication that the basis of their fear is real, and just needs confronting in order to "get used to the horror" or habituate to it. This is at odds with the cognitive understanding of anxiety, which seeks to guide the client to a discovery that the perception of threat was itself unfounded or exaggerated. Of course, there are times in therapy when the behavioural tasks or experiments feel foreboding, but in essence, the "face your fears" task is often best reframed as one of "choosing to find out how your world really works," recruiting the *curious* frame of mind of the client whenever possible. One very direct metaphor that may help in this regard is to refer to the *child who is scared of dogs* (clearly one should substitute a different animal/object if dogs happened to be the client's own focus of concern!) How would one help a child with such a fear? What would be most helpful for the child to grow up and become independent in a world inhabited also by dogs? Would the most helpful strategy be to shield the child from all possible contact with dogs? If not, why not? Would it be helpful to introduce the child to dogs but suggest the child always wear thick gloves and boots if ever in the vicinity of a dog? What might they discover if they were able to explore the world without such measures? And how might this help them? Often this discussion works particularly well when it concerns a named child well known to the client; the questions above then focus on that person.

Affective avoidance: "the stiff upper lip"

Safety-seeking behaviours in the form of avoidance often also occurs in the less obvious form of cognitive/affective avoidance. Trying to control emotions (usually because of the belief that one will be overwhelmed or otherwise damaged by their experience) is sometimes described by clients using their own metaphors; for example, being overwhelmed, swamped, swept away, and so on. Descriptions such as being frozen, being cut off, there being a plate of glass between oneself and the world are all common. An important step would be identifying the beliefs the person has about experiencing strong emotions and the role of such beliefs in motivating "covert" behaviours such as deliberate distraction. For example, one such behaviour might be depicted as "skating on thin ice" (verbally or in the person's own mind rushing ideas through their head so as not to dwell on them). Once identified, the person is helped to understand the way they prevent them from discovering that the things they fear do not happen.

Within-situation safety-seeking behaviours

While direct avoidance is the most obvious counterproductive strategy intended by the client to eliminate or reduce threat, the in-situation safety-seeking behaviour is its colourful partner in crime. These are strategies motivated by a desire to ward off or moderate the degree of threat, when the feared experience is (or has to be) encountered. For example, the panic client may sit down and hold onto a prop when they suspect they could be at risk of fainting, and the person with social phobia who fears they will run out of things to say and sound foolish may prepare a set of stock phrases to say in advance of a conversation and then monitor their own performance closely to check they are sounding OK. Unfortunately, safety-seeking behaviours prevent true disconfirmatory learning; that is, even though the feared outcome does not generally occur, the client is left attributing this benign outcome to the action of the safety behaviour, and builds no confidence whatsoever in the belief that they would have been OK anyway. The client inhabits a vulnerable world in which there is a narrow, fragile zone of safety, only to be found by playing slave to various arbitrary and limiting rules of behaviour.

To deal with this involves what is essentially a "leap of faith," where the client implicitly demonstrates their trust in the therapist by choosing to change the way they react to threat by confronting it in ways that can allow them to discover that the things they are afraid of do not happen. Implicitly or explicitly the concept of "leap of faith" is considered as part of therapy in preparation for behavioural experiments in which safety-seeking behaviours are dropped or reversed. If the person is to be asked to make a leap of faith, it is helpful if they can first reconsider and "loosen up" the basis of their threat beliefs, which motivate the safety-seeking and then be helped to understand why they are changing long-established patterns of behaviour in apparently risky ways. Several metaphors help develop insight into this process, and pave the way for behavioural experimentation outside of the grip of safety behaviours.

Particularly helpful is the story of the long-suffering *builder's apprentice*. In the town where one of the authors come from, builders play a trick on their new apprentice. They explain that the wall they are building is unstable until the cement between the bricks dries. The apprentice is asked to hold the wall to stop it from falling over. During the other workers' tea break, he stays there holding it, and sure enough, the wall stays up. The discussion then turns to whether there might be some similarity between this situation and anxiety-motivated behaviours for the client. How might it work? What are the consequences of keeping on doing these behaviours?

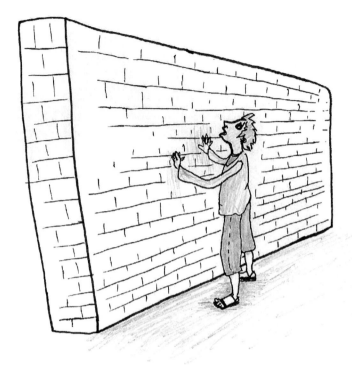

The metaphor is then extended by asking the client to consider how the builder's apprentice could have discovered that the wall was not going to fall. Sometimes this is done as a role-play, with the therapist taking the apprentice role and the client advising them. How is it possible to be sure that the wall won't fall? Usually the client will see that dropping the safety behaviour is the best means to work out what will happen. However, the apprentice might think that they were lucky this time, there was no breeze, so maybe next time the wall will fall. How could the apprentice do to check the *robustness* of the wall? How about giving it a push? What would the equivalent be for their anxiety-related fears? How can they "push the wall"?

A more lighthearted way of exploring the impact of safety-seeking behaviours is the story of the *elephants on the track*. The ticket collector notices an anxious-looking railway passenger ripping tiny pieces of paper up and throwing them out of the window onto the railway line. When asked why she is doing this she replies that it is to keep the elephants off the railway track. The ticket collector says he is puzzled; there are no elephants anywhere near the railway line. Of course, she replies, that's because I'm throwing pieces of paper out of the window. The client is asked if they can explain how she came to this conclusion. This type of humourous metaphor is helpful because it is both simple and amusing;

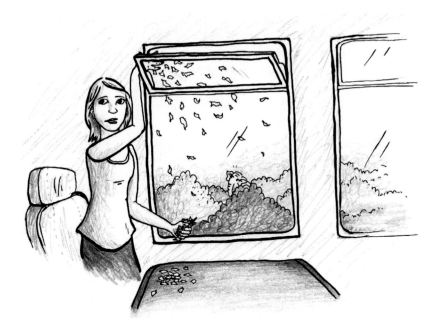

the humour can both offer the client some distance and also may further increase memorability. However, the therapist needs to make sure that they do not give the impression they are making light of the client's real concerns or attempts to help themselves. Indeed, it should be acknowledged that safety behaviours are a well-intentioned and often logical response to a belief in a genuine threat. However the therapist's principal task is to create a bridge in the client's mind between the elements of the metaphor and their own situation.

As mentioned in Chapter 3, when the client finds a metaphor, story, or other comparison funny, the therapist may need to help the client understand it even more to get at the core elements. A good way to do this is to ask *Why is that story funny?* and *Why does she continue to throw paper out the window?* In addition, it can be useful to crystallize the learning by a personification of the safety behaviour. *So the safety behaviour goes home with all the credit,* or *She is left at the mercy of the safety behaviour.*

Graded behaviours—"scaffolding on the building"

Confusion sometimes arises when therapists and clients jointly agree that inter-mediate behavioural steps, such as graded behaviours, are warranted to reach a particular goal. For example, a client wants to overcome their fear of heights, but feels they can only venture to the first floor of a building to begin with.

Or, a client wishes to overcome an obsession about contamination, but begins by removing their gloves only when in their own home, and not when on public transport. Are not such residual behaviours safety-seeking behaviours, and thus problematic? Or are they a natural human way of grading emotional responses and moving on a journey in the right direction?

The answer is that they could be either—the important distinction lies in the cognitions and intentions that underlie such behaviours. All may be well if the client recognizes that the "intermediate behaviour" is not the end-point, but that it is rather like *scaffolding on a building*—a helpful but not permanent structure to approach a rather daunting task in a manageable way. (A related metaphor is to liken the process to a child beginning to cycle with *stabilizers or trainer wheels*.) This may be a sensible and pragmatic option, especially if the client is otherwise likely to avoid the task completely, or to experience such an overwhelming emotional response that they risk dissociating. The implication is clear that the behaviour is not needed in the long run, and the natural next step will be to advance.

However, if the client holds onto a belief that their safety was, in fact, due to the implementation of this behaviour, or that taking the next step might be a "risk too far," then there may be a problem. Such a belief is suggestive of little cognitive shift and the behaviour may thus perpetuate the maintenance cycle of perceived threat. Metaphorically, this is back in the territory of the builder's apprentice, or the elephants on the track, described earlier. Finally, it should be noted that, even if the therapist has explicitly set up a graded task with the best of intentions and "scaffolding" rationale, there is a danger that the unwanted safety beliefs will nevertheless creep in. It is worth checking carefully to ensure this does not happen.

Disorder-specific factors

Figure 7.1 shows the cognitive model of the maintenance of anxiety disorders. Cognitive theory specifies that, over and above the general factors involved in anxiety becoming severe, disabling, and persistent, there are specific ones associated with particular diagnoses. This specificity arises from the meaning that lies at the heart of the maintenance model; the particular idiosyncratic meaning will be associated with particular experiences that prompt threat-related cognitions, the mixture of emotions that are driven, and the safety-seeking behaviours that are motivated. However, particular presentations/diagnoses are associated with particular types of meaning. Although the way research in CBT has been historically structured means that the specifics of our understanding of particular disorders tend to be couched in terms of psychiatric diagnoses, specificity is best regarded as dimensions and clusters of beliefs that are associated with (but not confined to) particular diagnoses at their most archetypal. Specific beliefs can and do straddle diagnostic groupings; beliefs may be disorder-specific (meaning that they typically occur in a particular disorder) and disorder relevant, so that a belief is not specific but nevertheless important. The overestimation of threat is disorder relevant across anxiety disorders; Table 7.1 shows disorder-specific belief domains for the anxiety disorders.

The focus of concern thus varies either in terms of gross differences (e.g. obsessive compulsive disorder being characterized by the interpretation of mental intrusions as a sign that the person may be responsible for harm to themselves or others—as opposed to panic disorder being characterized by the catastrophic misinterpretation of bodily/physiological sensations as a sign of some physical or mental disaster.) However, the distinctions can be more subtle, such as the distinction between panic disorder and health anxiety where in both instances the misinterpretation of bodily sensations is prominent but in panic but the feared catastrophe is regarded by the client as being imminent, that is within the next few seconds or minutes, as opposed to health anxiety where the feared catastrophe is located some months or years in the future. The implications of these differences are spelled out in the next section on a by disorder basis, summarized in Table 7.1.

Panic disorder

The central feature of panic disorder is the enduring tendency to misinterpret bodily sensations as a sign of impending (imminent) physical or mental catastrophe (Clark, 1986). Treatment involves identifying, from the careful description of a recent well-remembered panic, the panic vicious circle, examining evidence the person has for their catastrophic beliefs then actively testing these using carefully interwoven discussion and behavioural experiments. Discussion draws upon a range of metaphors both to aid the clients' understanding of how panic works and to help them understand the rationale for testing how best to deal with it.

Safety-seeking behaviours are almost always present; the builder's apprentice metaphor (see above) is extremely helpful in most panic clients as a way not only of explaining why their anxiety has persisted, but also as a general "softening up" as preparation for conducting behavioural experiments (in terms of "pushing the wall" as a way of conclusively discovering that the things they are afraid of are not going to happen). This generally applied metaphor is sometimes followed up by more specific examples focussed on particular catastrophic misinterpretations as a way of introducing particular behavioural experiments. For example, the client who fears suffocation and therefore usually tries to take extra breaths is prepared for a behavioural experiment

Table 7.1 Specific concerns and features of different anxiety disorders

Problem	Main focus of concern	Common safety-seeking behaviours	Other key features
Panic disorder	Catastrophic misinterpretation of anxiety-related bodily sensations as imminent danger	Seeking to control sensations and mental control	
Agoraphobia	As panic but also social concerns, fear of being trapped, abandoned	Avoidance of situations where a panic attack might occur, keep close to safety, talismans	Also occurs without panic e.g. in epilepsy, osteoporosis, irritable bowel syndrome
Health anxiety	Misinterpretation of bodily sensations/variations as indicating illness and suffering. Catastrophe not imminent. Also of health-related communications (doctors, Internet, media)	Reassurance-seeking, bodily checking, sometimes avoidance, seeks medical investigation and other information e.g. from Internet	Difficult to engage as some convinced basis of problem physical not psychological Also illness phobics ("I'm not ill now, but greatly fear for the future")
Generalized anxiety disorder	Overestimation of threat Intolerance of uncertainty Worry about worry	Rumination (e.g. to be prepared) Avoidance, procrastination, attention to potential threat ("scanning")	Sleep problems common
Obsessive compulsive disorder	Misinterpretation of intrusive thoughts, images, and impulses as indicating responsibility for serious harm to self or others	Washing, checking, neutralizing, thought suppression, reassurance seeking, avoidance	
Posttraumatic stress disorder	Re-experiencing symptoms (e.g. flashbacks, especially images) Continued ideas of threat, Sense of mental defeat	Thought suppression, avoidance of trigger (reminder) stimuli, withdrawal from others and activities, rumination	Memory for original trauma is fragmented and incomplete
Specific phobias	Ideas of imminent threat when confronted by feared stimulus Either/or the situation will be harmful; my response to the situation will be harmful	Avoidance of situations	
Social phobia	Misinterpretation of social situations as indicating that others are negatively evaluating them.	Avoid situations where they may have to do something in front of others, hide, self-monitor, put on a "front"	Often fear showing anxiety in social situations (e.g. shaking, blushing, sweating etc)

involving holding their breath (to see if they suffocate or not, and to discover that their body will "force" them to breathe). They are asked whether they have ever heard of anyone committing suicide by simply holding their breath. Why is this not possible? How do people breathe when they are swimming? Is it possible to hold your breath when swimming underwater, come up for one breath, back underwater, and so on?

Clients with panic problems are prone to self-monitor for internal signs of impending physical catastrophe. For example, they are able to detect slight fluctuations in heart rhythm, whereas other people would not be aware of this. Part of "decatastrophizing" is to help the person to understand that there is a clear alternative explanation for their sensitivity (rather than the idea that they are noticing more sensations because they have more as a result of there being something seriously physically wrong with them). It may be useful to suggest to them that their sensitivity to what is going on in their body can be best understood as a form of "special expertise." If someone is an expert on a subject, they tend to notice more details about that than others would. For example, what birds did you notice on your way here today? If you were an expert on birds, you would be able to provide names, etc. but others might just say "a brown one" (see *bird watcher* metaphor in greater detail on p. 134). The person with panic disorder can be thought of as an *expert on their own physical symptoms.*

Some clients have panic attacks during the night (nocturnal attacks). Perhaps this is less surprising when we think that our minds and bodies are still monitoring things and functioning in many respects during our sleep. For example, the client might be asked: Have you ever *woken at night needing the lavatory?* How did this happen? The conclusion is that we are aware of meaningful bodily sensations even when asleep. Threat is also perceived when asleep; for example, when (exhausted and sleep deprived) people have a new baby they may be able to sleep through loud outside noises, but *wake at very small baby noises.* Why is this? We are designed, to some extent, to be able to notice and monitor things that mean a lot to us.

Some clients with panic problems are concerned about the detrimental effects of stress on their heart. They might be asked: what's the most stressful job in the country? How have they survived? What about athletes, who have a faster acceleration of heart beats and for longer periods than anyone else? Panic clients often use implicit metaphors; they talk about the anxiety they have been experiencing "pushing them over the edge" and "taking me to snapping point."

The client who describes stress as being cumulative is invited to think about how they might be able to help the army with this information. Perhaps the army is training their special forces wrongly; instead of subjecting the soldiers to more and more difficult and stressful training, perhaps they should give the soldiers a long rest; after a year, maybe they will then be sufficiently destressed to carry out difficult missions? Why is this not true? What happens to those people as they go through their training? This effect can also be compared to training for a sporting event (e.g. the marathon). What happens over the course of training?

Obsessive compulsive disorder

An important component in treating obsessive compulsive disorder (OCD) is identifying the beliefs that motivate the client's compulsive behaviour. However, in some chronic cases where the client has stopped resisting their compulsions, these meanings have dropped from awareness; the person simply washes or checks in particular situations, with no apparent awareness of motivating beliefs. To help them understand what has happened (and how the beliefs can be better identified), the therapist can use a type of metaphor that illustrates the motivation for "proceduralized" or overpracticed behaviours. In the client who drives, the therapist says: "This reminds me of something which happens when we drive. What do you do when you come to a red traffic light?" When the client says "I stop" the therapist asks them why they stop. Usually the response is "I just do". But, persists the therapist, "What is the real reason? "What will happen if you don't stop?" It is identified that not stopping might result in injury or even death for the driver and others, that the car will be wrecked, the police might prosecute and so on. The therapist follows up by saying "OK, so is that what goes through your mind at a red traffic light? No? But are we agreed that this is your motivation....at the back of your mind? I wonder if your OCD is similar?" In discussion, it is considered that there may be fears at the back of the person's mind when they ritualize; how can they find out what those fears are? The client is returned to the traffic lights metaphor... "Supposing I was an unethical researcher who wanted to confirm what your fears are in relation to stopping at a red light. What kind of experiment could I do? How about I tamper with your brakes? What do you think would flash through your mind when you found your car rushing towards the busy junction?" This is followed up by "Let's go back to your rituals. Using the same principle, how could we find out what fears lie behind these?" Typically the client will suggest that they might try not to ritualize in order to see what fears then appear. Note that this "assessment experiment" has been suggested by the client rather than the therapist; the rationale for it is already clear, and the client rather than the therapist has initiated behaviour change. The therapist's role is then to help the client to set up and record the results of this experiment. For further discussion on automaticity in cognitive processes see Chapter 5, p. 79.

A range of metaphors are applied in OCD to help the client make alternative sense of their experiences, to help them find out that far from preventing harm and distress OCD causes and increases their anxiety and discomfort and takes over their life. For many clients the history of onset of OCD suggests that it began in the guise of a "concerned friend," suggesting to them that they should take precautions against harm. Often they still see it in this way despite the damage it has done to their life. OCD is personified; it says to the client "All you need to do is wash when you feel contaminated, that will make you feel better". However, the therapist suggests, perhaps it has now become a *bully*. The comparison is developed further; how does a bully work? What do they want? The aim is to conclude that the bully makes their victim do things for them against their will. The client is asked about what advice they might offer a child (usually asking the client to choose a specific child as part of the discussion.....their son, niece, godchild). The child says "Please can you give me some money? I need it to give to the big boy at school. He said that he would hit me if I don't get him some money today." The client is asked "would you give him the money? Why not? What advice would you give him?" As the discussion is developed, the idea of confronting the bully/OCD is developed. How does this apply to their OCD? Later in therapy, the metaphor is used to further develop longer term strategies. If the bully says to do a particular thing, you might consider doing the exact opposite; that's what you need to do with the OCD. As an alternative to a bully, OCD can be compared to a manipulative liar who tries to make you do what it wants rather than what you want.

Another metaphor helpful in understanding the "big picture" in terms of OCD is to compare it to an addiction. The OCD client is asked to consider what someone who is addicted to a drug feels about their next "fix." Often, they will think "the only thing that can make me better is to take the drug." This may be true, but for how long? What is the longer term effect of having yet another "hit"? What will happen in the longer term? Here the aim is to help the client see that the short-term "benefits" of ritualizing are more than outweighed by the longer term tendency to need more and more. This is often described by the phrase "the solution has become the problem."

Another metaphorical way to explain the counter productive role of obsessional behaviour is the idea of *Digging to get out of a hole* (see also Chapter 4, p. 61). OCD involves trying too hard, and sometimes the client feels that they should find better ways of being obsessional. The client often wants to find out from an expert about how to be a "better and more efficient" obsessional; it is pointed out to them that no one ever got rid of obsessional worries using compulsive behaviour. For example, a client with contamination fears suggests that they might worry less if a surgeon taught them how to wash their hands more effectively. The therapist asks them to consider the possibility that they are not only digging to get out of a hole, but also that they are under the impression that they will get out of the hole if they improved their digging technique and had a better or bigger spade. The function of reassurance and the involvement of others in rituals or avoidance can be described in the same type of way; will having a friend come into the hole you are digging and to dig as well be helpful?

Once the obsessional client has understood that there may be a different way of thinking about what is happening to them (for example, that their problem is not that they are contaminated, but that they are worried about being contaminated; that their problem is not that they are going to kill their child, but rather that they love their child so much that they are preoccupied by worries about harming them), they need to progress to "choosing to change." The therapist can convey their understanding of how difficult this is for the client by referring to them taking a *leap of faith* by enduring their fears; the client is reminded that it would be frightening but immensely worthwhile in the longer term to go against "the bully."

Sometimes, clients say that they would like to choose to change, but it seems to them to be "too risky." This is particularly likely for those who feel that not ritualizing will result in an extremely serious catastrophe, such as the death of a loved one. The person (understandably) says that they cannot take even the smallest risk in this case. This can be focussed on using the *insurance metaphor*. The therapist says "When you talk about covering risk, that reminds me of insurance, which is all about risk. Let's think about your house insurance; does it cover all risks? How about the risk of terrorist attacks? Acts of God? If you are negligent?" The discussion should reveal that not all risks are covered. The therapist follows this discussion with "Well, I think you would want to make sure that you were covered for all these risks. I'm going to offer you a new insurance policy which covers all of those things not covered by your present policy. Would you like that?" When the client agrees they would, then the therapist says "OK; the first premium is two million pounds. Do you still want it? Why not?" The client indicates in some way that it is too expensive, and the therapist responds by saying "You know, that kind of reminds me of your OCD! I know that you want to make sure that you don't take any risks at all, and that OCD for you is a kind of insurance, but have you considered what the *costs* are?"

This is followed by a potentially distressing discussion of the range of "costs" of their OCD. What has it cost them in terms of their happiness? The impact on their family? And so on, including the reality of how OCD has affected them. What the use of this metaphor does is help the client take a different perspective on what is happening to them. Note that this perspective is also normalizing. The therapist might point out that anyone, including themselves, who believes that they can prevent terrible things from happening by performing a simple and brief neutralizing action (a check, a wash, a prayer) would do so. However, in OCD, it's not brief, over and done with. It's washing now, and again, and again, today, tomorrow, the next day, next week, next month, next year, and so on for the rest of your life, with the cost mounting all the time without making any real difference to risk. Clients who are still struggling with the "leap of faith" might be asked to consider what they would like to achieve in their life, in terms of goals etc. (see Chapter 5, p. 96). What would they like their obituary to say: "She was very clean? She checked a lot?" This point is related back to the idea of cost of their obsessional behaviour and the way OCD prevents them from achieving the things they want, such as having a family, going on holiday, having a good relationship with their friends and family and so on.

Later in therapy when things are going well (especially in clients with long-standing problems), it is common for many clients to hesitate about continuing therapy; they explain this as being that they don't want to *rock the boat*. They seem to have reached a *plateau*, and seem to wish to stay there rather than continue on up, perhaps because they fear the consequences of doing this. Note that these are implicit metaphors. What the client usually means is that, after many years of suffering from crippling OCD, they have made considerable progress, and are better than they have been for many years. They therefore fear that if they do more (rock the boat) that this might result in them losing the gains they have made. Best therefore to stop at this point and enjoy how things are now without further risk. They feel that they should not *tempt fate* by doing the yet more challenging things which might be needed for them to progress further.

Two metaphors can be helpful here. The first is directly derived from the client's own description of *rocking the boat*. In the past, the therapist says, you were right not to rock the boat, because you were at the mercy of your OCD. Before therapy began, the client only felt able to survive by taking care not to rock the boat, which felt like it was out on the high seas, being tossed around with the constant risk of being overwhelmed and "drowned" by their anxiety. However, since that time things have changed hugely. As they have engaged in therapy, they have been able to steer the boat much closer to the coastline than before. Although the client is still in the boat, what have they discovered about the water? How deep is it now? Is the cost of "rocking the boat" actually much lower than it was before? While it was understandable to huddle in the boat and not disturb it in deep water, perhaps the water is only inches deep now.

If this is true, then the client needs to rock the boat so that it capsizes and lets them out. If they do that, then they will be able to walk to the shore. When they reach the shore, they can then get on with their life, and enjoy the benefits of not being stuck in the boat. The client is asked to consider the possibility that not rocking the boat is now part of the problem rather than the solution.

The second useful metaphor is also for when clients express doubts about *finishing the job*. Do they really need to go any further? Why not just stop therapy now that things are so much better? This is compared to having an infected wound. The wound has been cleaned, the dirt taken out, and antiseptic applied. However, there is still a small infected area, and it looks like it would be painful to clean that out. Maybe it would be better just to leave it be, put a bandage over it and hope for the best? The client is asked to consider the wisdom of doing that; usually they say that this is a bad idea, as the infection would simply re-spread, and the previous good work of cleaning and disinfecting would be undone. Maybe, the therapist says, it is the same with the residual OCD fears?

At this point in therapy, the client has usually made considerable changes, and the main threat to completing treatments and getting completely "cured" is the client's feeling that they can usefully reach a compromise with the OCD (note again the implicit metaphor, making OCD an entity). This means that the client runs the risk of sustaining their OCD at a more subtle level rather than eradicating it. This strategy is compared to another situation; for the religious person, can be compared to making a *pact with the devil*. Can you have only a little pact with the devil? A similar metaphor involves comparing it to corruption: if you only take a small bribe, is that OK? Why not?

Health anxiety

The essential component of severe and persistent health anxiety (diagnostically referred to as "hypochondriasis," a term almost universally disliked by clients, and itself a metaphor, in this case the "wandering stomach" or hypochondrium) is preoccupation with the fear of having, and belief that one may have, a serious, usually life-threatening, illness. Health anxiety shares characteristics of both panic disorder and OCD, in that the misinterpretation of bodily variations is prominent (having an impact on selective attention and physiological factors, including acuity as illustrated by the *bird watcher* example earlier, p. 134), with the delayed time course (relative to panic) making it more like OCD, with reassurance seeking and checking being prominent.

As already described for anxiety disorders in general, the initial focus is on the generation of an alternative, less threatening account of the person's anxiety and preoccupation. The development of a *vicious flower* type model as a shared understanding is the appropriate starting point. Given that the time course of the feared illness is usually far in the future, it is important to emphasize evidence for the cognitive formulation rather than seeking disconfirmation of the person's fears. The *insurance metaphor* described earlier for OCD (p. 146) is an important engagement tool when clients take the view that they must check, seek reassurance, and medical investigation because they are unable to tolerate the risk if they do not do so.

Also prominent is the seeking of medical information, directly through doctors and medical tests/investigations and indirectly through reading and the Internet. Some of the most specific metaphors relate to helping the person to deal with this aspect of the problem. Identifying the need for medical reassurance as similar to an *addiction* can be helpful (see p. 145, this chapter). Selective attention metaphors described earlier are also important.

Social phobia

Social phobia involves the fear of negative evaluation by other people. Situations that provoke social anxiety can vary widely, and may include eating or writing in public view, engaging in and/or maintaining conversation with one or more people, or public speaking. The central characteristics are a fear that one will do or say something to cause embarrassment, and a belief that others will judge one's performance critically. The Clark and Wells (1995) model allows a parsimonious cognitive conceptualization that integrates negative beliefs about one's likely performance and others' likely reactions, physiological manifestations of anxiety, safety behaviours designed to reduce the social threat, and a tendency to focus attention inwardly upon oneself. In addition, anticipatory and postevent rumination are common, which exacerbate the problem. The interaction of these processes helps explain the maintenance of social phobia, and the lack of habituation of social fears commonly seen (or not seen!) over a period of many years.

One important concept, in working with social phobia, is the important notion that generally speaking, one does not outwardly appear as anxious as one feels. Frequently, at the outset of therapy, clients with social phobia really believe their feelings are highly visible for all to see. They may feel that they sweat profusely, tremble uncontrollably, blush as red as a tomato, or look like nervous gibbering wrecks. They feel vulnerable and *transparent*, as if there is no barrier between their inner feelings and the outside world. Others, they fear, can and will instantly see through them, see their anxieties and judge them as weak. Cognitive therapy can assist in providing corrective information about the degree to which one's feelings really show through. One powerful technique is video feedback, in which the client watches themselves objectively on video, typically having engaged in a short role-play (e.g. a social conversation) under moderate anxiety conditions. They contrast how they predicted they would come across with the objective reality on the video. Commonly, there are major discrepancies, allowing the client to build confidence in the belief that not all their anxiety is visible, and a neutral observer would not see through them—*they are not a glass box.*

This glass box metaphor can be developed or extended in several ways. One client ran with the notion of the glass box, and said he realized that he had previously always felt like he was living in a *fish tank* (transparent, and for everyone to gaze at). Now, he realized *he* was the one who had been doing all the gazing. This insightful observation relates to another central theme in cognitive therapy for social phobia, that of self-focussed attention. Clients often spend a great deal of time self-monitoring, studying, and criticizing their own performance—but they project this activity onto other people, usually in spite of precious little evidence that others scrutinize or judge them. For clients with social phobia, "living in their heads" is doing them no favours; it fills their minds with their worst fears and self-impressions. With appropriate sensitivity, it may therefore be valuable to point this out directly: "Your head is a dangerous place to be—we need you to get *out of your head and into the world!*"

The transformatory metaphor of getting out of your head and into the world encourages an attentional shift from a self-focussed perspective to an externally focussed perspective, which will often have an anxiety-reducing effect right away. However, this is not merely a useful trick. A key function of the external attentional shift is in data gathering—to allow the client access to a wealth of information about how they are really seen by others. For example, a brief glance at other people, while externally attending, will determine how many of them are actually staring, or looking critically. A wide variety of behavioural experiments may be conducted, with the common thread of gathering valuable data about how others see them. A useful metaphor here can be one of *tuning in to a radio station.* Previously, the client with social phobia spent much time either avoiding social situations, or engaging but being self-focussed. Therefore, their heads were full of noise, and they were not tuned in. They had no access to the information that was important for them to hear—how others really viewed them.

Another component of cognitive therapy for social phobia involves what Adrian Wells has called *broadening the bandwidth.* This involves shaking up and purposefully breaking and experimenting with some of the rather rigid rules of conduct that people with social phobia have constructed for themselves. For example, clients may operate according to the rule *I can only speak to someone else if it lasts no more than two minutes and I am sitting down* or

I must come across as ultra-laid back and like I am knowledgeable about current affairs and witty. Often such "rules for living" represent a codification of how safety behaviours are used, which in turn stem from the core fears that the individual possesses (e.g. running out of things to say, looking shaky, being seen as anxious, stupid, boring, etc). The result is a *narrowing* of behaviour patterns, almost like the person is "walking a tightrope" of behavioural rules, such that any deviation may result in social disaster. This metaphor is valuable in capturing the vulnerability, anxiety, and restriction experienced by people with social phobia. It also paves the way for a purposeful set of experiments designed to explore their social world more fully.

Posttraumatic stress disorder

Posttraumatic stress disorder (PTSD) is a response to an overwhelming traumatic event, observed in a proportion of people who have endured or witnessed such an event. Involuntary and distressing re-experiencing of the original memory trace is the hallmark feature of PTSD, accompanied by avoidance and numbing symptoms and persistent hyperarousal. Several models of PTSD have been described (e.g. Brewin & Holmes, 2003). One of the most comprehensive is that of Ehlers and Clark (2000), which centres its formulation around the persistent sense of "current threat" observed in people with PTSD. Three main factors account for the maintenance of this illusory sense of threat: a memory trace that is easily triggered via low-level sensory stimuli and not adequately contextualized within autobiographical memory ("unprocessed" in shorthand; see also Chapter 5, p. 84); a set of idiosyncratic negative appraisals relating to the trauma itself and/or the effects of the trauma; and a set of behavioural response strategies that are understandable but counterproductive, typically including attempts to suppress the memory and its associated emotions, avoidance of places, people and activities connected with the trauma, and rumination about one or more issues relating to the trauma (e.g. "Why me?").

In PTSD work, there is a need to characterize the peculiar nature of the traumatic memory, which behaves as if it has freshly occurred, is triggered easily into consciousness outside of the client's control, and is in a raw, emotional, fragmented state, undulled by the passage of time. Furthermore, there is a need to socialize the client to the rather abstract idea that this memory will behave more like an ordinary "bad" memory if some time is spent processing it carefully in conscious awareness. Metaphors are an ideal way to convey these concepts.

One metaphor here is the *overfull kitchen cupboard* (though there are many variants on this; see Chapter 2, p. 15 and Chapter 5, p. 151). The cupboard (representing memory) is generally organized and orderly, with the doors shut. If an item is required, the door is carefully opened and the piece selected. This corresponds to a memory being accessed voluntarily. In trauma, however, there is repetitive involuntary activation of the memory. This is like suddenly, out of the blue, someone thrusts a giant mass of kitchen crockery into your hands, shouting *Stow them away, quick!* You try to shove them into the kitchen cupboard but the items do not fit; there is a tumble of crockery, the doors fly open, and the items spill out of the cupboard. You try again hurriedly to stuff the items away, and the same happens, again and again. What needs to be done to resolve this repetitive cycle? Of course, the pieces need to be taken out, gone through carefully, organized and finally put back in an orderly way in the cupboard.

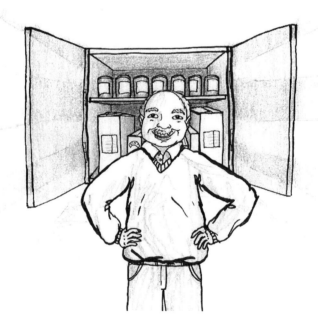

A simple variant on this, also incorporating the notion of memory fragmentation, is the *jigsaw with pieces everywhere*. Everywhere you step, in whichever direction, you tread on jigsaw pieces. Closing your eyes is no good, and neither is trying to forget about the jigsaw. You keep treading on pieces. The solution? To spend some careful time sorting and reconstructing the jigsaw, so it will finally fit in its box, and the lid close. Sometimes clients will, in popular jargon, speak of trying to "put a lid on the box," often realizing they have not been able to, by means of avoidance and suppression. The jigsaw metaphor may be a

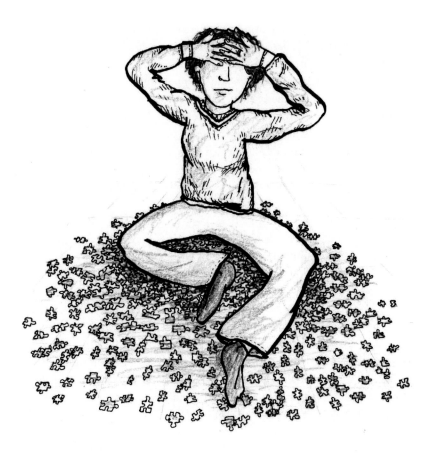

helpful elaboration of this, introducing a basic explanatory component and a basic rationale for memory processing.

Another powerful metaphor here is linked to some elementary neuroscience, requires little *actual* understanding of neuroscience, and can be therapeutically destigmatizing, especially for those who have questioned their sanity, having symptoms of PTSD. It describes the workings of the *amygdala and hippocampus*, and may be shared with the client as follows (with the aid of a diagram):

Therapist: There's a lot of research going on into how the brain works, and although much is still not known, two parts seem really important in coding memories during trauma. The amygdala has very fast connections with the senses, like sight, sound and smell. It lays down a memory which is sensory and emotional. Now one of its jobs is a bit like being *a guard dog*—so if something looks, smells or sounds a bit like the trauma (e.g. you hear a siren) then the amygdala "barks", sending "red alert" messages to the rest of your brain, bringing images to mind and making you jumpy and distressed. It's basically fast, and essential for survival, but it's not terribly clever. Then there's another bit of your brain, the hippocampus, which stores the context of what's happening, a kind of story which includes what happened, when, and what it all meant. This is slower to operate but is cleverer. This is a bit like the *dog's owner*. When the whole system is working properly, the two parts (guard dog and its owner) communicate well. So for example when a siren is heard, the guard dog may be about to bark but the owner sends a reassuring signal, sort of 'It's OK, this siren is different, the trauma is not going to happen again'. Does that make sense so far?

Client: Yes I think so.

Therapist: OK, but the trouble in PTSD is that these two bits aren't communicating as they should. It's like for this particular memory, your hippocampus isn't wired up properly to the amygdala. Therefore, when you encounter any sights or sounds which are trauma triggers, the amygdala barks, and it's like a dog without its owner. It's not its fault, it doesn't know any better. But it can't get what's going on in any context.

Client: So, why is that—why is it not wired up properly?

Therapist: That's a good question. It may be that because the trauma was so intense an emotional experience, the priority for your brain was for the amygdala to do its job, to get you safe, and less resource was there to lay down the wiring bit.

Client: So how does that help me—what can be done?

Therapist: Well, if you like, there's nothing basically wrong with the dog, or its owner, but the dog needs more training. In other words, there's nothing wrong with your amygdala or hippocampus, but we really need to get them communicating about the trauma properly. So that means we need to tell the story and allow the emotions to get triggered, but we do it carefully so that the system gets wired up properly.

Otto (2000) describes a close relative of this metaphor, in the idea of the "limbic kid"—a frightened child who cannot adequately discriminate between a cue which resembles danger and one which is actually dangerous. There are also a number of simpler variants on the "barking dog" amygdala metaphor, particularly when looking at the hypervigilance aspects of PTSD. One would be to consider the system as an *oversensitive alarm*. The alarm keeps going off (jumpiness, emotional arousal triggered by innocuous stimuli) and the alarm is very loud and well-designed so that attempts to block your ears, turn away, disconnect it or disable it will fail. (Indeed, many house alarms don't stop ringing even if you pull them off the wall and walk down the road with them, apparently). Therefore, the solution is that the system needs to be reset. Lots of experimentation may be required to test out and reset the alarm so it does not trigger so much at innocuous events.

People who have been traumatized may benefit from some early assertive action to reclaim their life (Ehlers & Clark, 2000). Trauma has a way of making people feel completely stuck, frozen in time, as if they are living in a time warp and nothing can move on. Furthermore, trauma can instigate a paralyzing effect on important parts of the individual's life across several domains including work, leisure, and personal relationships. Two metaphorical personifications can be helpful here. First, the trauma memory can be given agency, metaphorically—it's the *"memory talking."* It can be elaborated that part of the stuckness, the "frozen in time" feeling is due to characteristics of the trauma memory. Having this phrase to hand can offer a simple but powerful metaphorical maneuvre. It succinctly reminds the client of the theory of trauma memories, it helps reduce the sense of craziness that many clients with PTSD experience, and it can instill a hope of change, rather than stuckness, as a principal task of therapy is to assist by processing the trauma memory.

Second, the trauma itself can be "personified." *Trauma is like a robber*—as if the event wasn't terrible enough, the trauma has tried to steal away other parts of your old life—e.g. you used to go out regularly, use transport with impunity, etc. and now this is all gone. So, we need to reclaim some parts of your old life once again. We need to "show the trauma" that it won't be allowed to steal all of those things. Even if it takes some while to reclaim, and not everything may look exactly the same, we can start reclaiming some things right away. This metaphor obviously needed highly individual tailoring, and exploration of what the first steps could be in reclaiming one's life. Particular sensitivity will be needed where there has been real permanent change, for example, if someone has lost a loved one, or lost a limb. However, this simple metaphor can be hugely empowering, and sow the seeds of assertive action, which can be so needed in someone who has been traumatized or feels cast into the role of a victim.

Generalized anxiety disorder

There are several viable cognitive theories of generalized anxiety disorder (GAD), all of which emphasize the importance of overestimation of threat and the role of worry. Beck, Emery, and Greenberg (1985) emphasize negative appraisals in terms of probability, "awfulness," coping and rescue factors (see p. 128, this chapter). Borkovec and Wells both emphasize the importance of worry, particularly strategic (deliberate/voluntary) components; Borkovec suggested that worry was a type of experiential avoidance; in particular, he hypothesized that worry tended to damp down frightening imagery (Borkovec & Inz, 1990). More recently he has emphasized the importance of interpersonal factors and acceptance. Wells (2000) labelled worry processes in terms of metacognitive beliefs, with two distinct types being specified: beliefs in the benefits of worry (e.g. "worrying keeps me safe by warning me about what can go wrong") and negative beliefs about worry (e.g. "If I keep on worrying like this and losing sleep, I will go mad"). Freeston, Rheaume, Letarte et al. (1994) have emphasized intolerance of uncertainty as key; if the person is uncertain, they defensively assume that the worst will happen. The role of worry can be explained as being like being caught up in a *whirlwind*; negative ideas chase each other round, catching the hapless client up in the middle, swept along without seeming to be able to control things.

Meares and Freeston (2008) describe excessive worrying as analogous to a *problem of traffic flow*. Worry operates as a stream of thoughts and images, which spirals out of control. In the same way, therefore, that it would be fruitless to attempt to solve a traffic congestion problem by honing in on the motion of one particular car, likewise overly focussing on one particular worry does not address the systemic problem of worrying. Congestion in one place will often "spread" to other neighboring roads, and worries will often spread and jump from one topic to another. Driving rules influence traffic flow, and overarching worry rules (e.g. *Worrying will help me work out what to do*) influence the process of worrying. Worriers are often highly focussed on the *content* of the worry of the moment, and this metaphor helps with an important shift to a recognition that the *process* of worry needs addressing.

A key difficulty faced by people who worry to a pathological extent is the intolerance of uncertainty. While a restricted class of future events are predictable, such as the sun rising and setting, or the trains being crowded at rush hour, a great many future events are inherently unpredictable and outcomes uncertain. At the mundane end of things, buses may not run on time, and people may be late for work. At the more severe end of things, cities may suffer earthquakes and trains might crash. We can speculate hypothetically about the future, we can ignore the future and deal with things as they occur, or we can worry extensively about the future.

Intolerance of uncertainty may be thought of as an *allergy* (Dugas & Robichaud, 2006). Most people are familiar with the idea that a tiny quantity of allergic substance (e.g. a single nut, to someone with a nut allergy) is sufficient to trigger a severe and sometimes life-threatening reaction in the sufferer. Likewise, a powerful worry reaction can be triggered in someone when a *seed of doubt* is planted in their minds—even if the uncertainty is negligible by other people's standards—such as a 1 in 1000 chance of a car breaking down because it's running low on petrol.

Summary

In this chapter, a range of metaphors have been outlined, some which are applicable across a wide range of disorders and others which are more specifically relevant to particular diagnoses. We have emphasized the importance of understanding before we seek to be understood. In anxiety disorders, clients by definition experience extremely high levels of fear and threat; in treatment we seek to help them see that their fears may not be justified and that they can therefore choose to change. In doing so, we ask extraordinary things of people who are in states of fear or even terror; confront your fears, trust me, "feel the fear and do it anyway" and so on. Throughout, we must make sure we justify the way we ask people to trust us. The skilful and collaborative use of metaphor as described in this chapter can help the client to understand why they should take the apparently horrendous risks that we require of them. Embedding the use of metaphor in the context of a shared understanding of a different, less threatening narrative of how the person's particular anxiety problem affects them can help them to take the "leap of faith," which is required to discover how their world really works. "Trust me" is not a right, but should be earned.

Chapter 8

Bipolar disorders and mood swings

Introduction

Whatever their diagnosis, many of our clients experience mood swings that they may find hard to explain, difficult to control, and lead to significant problems. People who fit the criteria for bipolar disorder have had severe and enduring swings in mood (mania or hypomania and depression) that can have a huge impact on relationships and their working life, typically entailing hospital admission and medication (see later). Yet, during some of their high moods, people with bipolar disorder may feel at their most productive, creative, and sociable. Therefore, clients are often ambivalent about these experiences—recognizing both the extremely positive and the threatening qualities of the mood states. Clients with other diagnoses, such as borderline personality disorder, schizoaffective disorder, and alcohol or substance abuse, can also report similar experiences. It may come as no surprise that these individuals often strive to understand why they experience such chaotic and conflicting feelings, why they impact so much on other people, and why many of their moods seem to be out of their control.

Cognitive therapy for bipolar disorder and mood swings can help clients to develop an understanding of their mood, manage it better, and move their life forward despite these problems (Mansell, Morrison, Reid, Lowens, & Tai, 2007). Most clients will already be taking psychotropic medication prior to beginning CBT, yet typically CBT is offered as an additional intervention, or sometimes for those who do not take medication for various reasons.

In the search for self-understanding, metaphors can be invaluable. In this section, we will introduce some examples of metaphors that have been used to understand the mood swings that often characterize bipolar disorders and related problems. We will cover a mixture of therapist-generated and client-generated metaphors that have proved useful in CBT. Then, we will spend some time articulating one narrative metaphor that may be particularly helpful for both clients and therapists in trying to understand and validate the lived experience and history of a person with a bipolar disorder.

Bipolar disorders

Bipolar disorders are characterized by periods of high and low moods that differ widely in presentation. Classically clients have had periods of mania and depression in the past and are vulnerable to relapses in the future; this is known as bipolar I disorder. While bipolar depression overlaps with the features of unipolar depression with some minor exceptions (Mansell, Colom, & Scott, 2005), mania is a diverse and often chaotic state of mind. Mania is characterized by at least a week of either euphoric or irritable mood, alongside a range of experiences indicating high "activation," including racing thoughts, distractibility, feeling rested after limited sleep, and talking so fast that it is hard to interrupt (pressure of speech). In studies of phenomenology, many other experiences are also reported during mania including depressed mood, anxiety, and paranoia (Mansell & Pedley, 2008). At its extreme, people experience psychosis during mania, engage in high-risk activities that are out of character (e.g. promiscuous behaviour; spending large amounts of money), and are often hospitalized. Even outside an episode of depression or mania, people with bipolar disorder often have compromised lives, continuing to find it hard to return to work and maintain good relationships.

Despite the apparent extremes of bipolar I disorder, many people with bipolar disorders who seek psychological therapy may have had long periods of apparent wellness. Others, who fit the criteria for bipolar II disorder, will have experienced depression and hypomania—a briefer or milder period of high mood through which they can manage their lives, or may even excel in creativity or productivity. It is becoming clear that the classification of bipolar disorders may be unhelpful for several reasons (Mansell & Pedley, 2008). For example, bipolar disorder is defined historically—through having episodes in the past—and so someone with a diagnosis is never truly "recovered." Also, many people with problematic mood swings do not fit the established categories, or switch between them over time. Thus, given similar issues in other classes of disorders such as the eating disorders (Fairburn, Cooper, & Shafran, 2003), a fruitful way to approach delivering CBT is to work on the phenomenon of mood swings itself, which transcends diagnostic category, rather than any specific bipolar disorder diagnosis (Mansell et al., 2007).

Client metaphors

The key focus of people with bipolar disorder seems to be their "feelings," or more precisely, their "internal state." One focus is mood—which ranges widely from extremely low, self-critical and suicidal, to extremely high, exuberant and "expansive." Some people talk about the state of their mind—whether their thoughts are "cloudy," "muddled," or slowed down, or whether they are the opposite—"racing" through their head like they can't "keep up the pace." At other times, they describe a state within their body—either lifeless and weighed down, or highly agitated, restless, and "buzzing." The way anyone describes internal states seems to be ripe for metaphors, maybe because we are trying to put across a perception we are having that no one else can experience for themselves. We need to resort to concepts or entities "out there" to try to describe them. Even the ideas of high-versus-low mood, ups-and-downs in mood, and mood "swings" are metaphorical as they are based on properties of physical objects. Thus, one can almost not escape from metaphor when working with these issues.

Within cognitive models of bipolar disorder (e.g. Bentall, 2003; Mansell et al., 2007; Jones, 2001), the meanings of internal states are critical because they are seen to drive behaviour that further impacts on mood and the social environment. Within the integrative cognitive model (Mansell et al., 2007), it is the conflicting and extreme personalized appraisals of internal states that are seen to drive mood swings. For example, an individual may believe that their highs are both the only way they know to achieve extreme success and overcome all their problems *and* a state that is likely to lead to loss of control, conflict with others, and mental breakdown. Within the model, CBT is directed to help people to resolve these conflicting beliefs and build on their personal goals in a way that is less contingent upon their mood. Thus, during CBT, it is important both to help the client gain an awareness of the internal states they experience, and to distil the meanings that they attach to them, both positive and negative. Again, metaphors seem to be a natural way of exploring these perceptions and appraisals.

Table 8.1 provides a range of examples of clients' own metaphors about internal states that encapsulate their meanings. They have been divided into the domains of internal states—affective, physiological, cognitive, and behavioural—and contrasted into states of high and low activation, consistent with the integrative cognitive model. The domains of internal states are not meant to be precise, but give a flavour of the kinds of internal states that attract extreme personal meanings in bipolar disorder. The therapy dialogue below illustrates the way that one client described how her low feelings begin:

Therapist: So you get this feeling when you've completed a project. What is it?
Client: It's like a drop. It just feels like a drop.
Therapist: Is there any other way you can describe this drop feeling?
Client: Like an empty drop... I don't know. It's just an empty drop.
Therapist: An emptiness?

Client: Yeah.

Therapist: Is that pretty distressing?

Client: Yes, it makes me think I just don't want to do anything or go anywhere.

Therapist: OK, so we have the empty drop feeling and then this thought that you don't want to do anything or go anywhere?

Client: That's right.

There are several reasons why it can be helpful to elicit metaphorical descriptions of internal states. First, it can help the client to become aware of the internal state itself, as a separate process from their appraisal of the state. This helps to build a formulation where feelings and thoughts are separable. Second, while the client is describing the internal state, they are experiencing it typically from a detached perspective rather than one that is immersed in the feeling or avoidant of it. In this way, it may already help the person to start to tolerate a wider bandwidth of feelings and begin to interrupt the mood-appraisal-behaviour cycle that is thought to maintain or escalate mood symptoms.

Table 8.1 Client's metaphors for internal states that encapsulate their personal meanings

Activation	Domain	Metaphor example	Encapsulated meaning
High	Affective	"Souris"—meaning the "mouse" and the "smile"	Happiness means being cute, and excitable but also the centre of other people's attention
	Physiological	"Buzzing like a bee"	Sensation of arousal has a buzzing quality that is energizing yet entails frenetic activity
	Cognitive	"Quicksilver" thinking	Fast, bright and efficient thinking that is very hard to control
	Behavioural	The Hulk	Bursting with energy to gain strength and power to save people in distress yet becoming ugly and frightening in the process
Low	Affective	Blackness	A feeling devoid of any emotional "colour"
	Physiological	"Empty drop" feeling at the pit of stomach	A serious loss associated with low mood; feeling "gutted"
	Cognitive	Cotton wool	Thoughts that are ineffectual and very difficult to "catch"
	Behavioural	Huddled into a ball	A low feeling that one is ashamed of, and a need to avoid attention

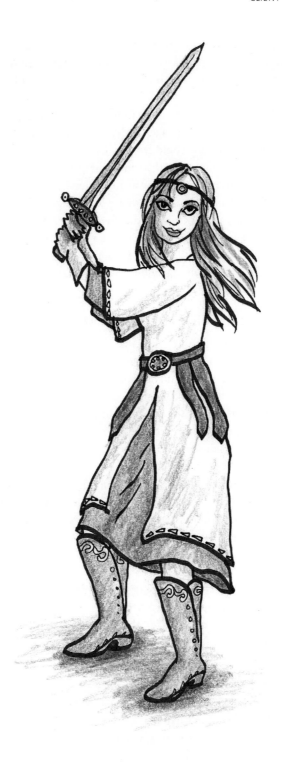

Third, the therapist can use the metaphor with clients subsequently because it may be more memorable than a vague, less personalized description of an internal state. This can promote validation and also potential change strategies.

For example, the client who equated feeling low with being *huddled into a ball* clearly had a very negative image of what her low mood was like. She was asked to imagine whether she could feel low in any other way. Could she feel low and be sitting in a chair rather than huddled? Has she ever experienced this? Would this be a more acceptable way to feel low? The client who used the metaphor of *The Hulk* to express the paradox of her high energy states as both powerful but frightening worked with the therapist to imagine an alternative image of her high energy states. The image of a "warrior princess" provided this alternative. It represented a side of her that was more consistent and sophisticated in her use of energy and that did not unintentionally frighten others with her behaviour.

Highs and lows as 'flipsides of the same coin'

Moving on from the metaphors for specific internal states, we can explore the meaning of both high and low internal states in relation to one another. It has long been suggested that mania and depression are both defensive reactions to the same underlying "complex" (Abraham, 1911). Within the integrative cognitive model, this is also partly the case in that the cycles that drive low or high mood tend to take people away from the normal experience of emotional processing that accompanies dealing with long-term distressing problems; the cycles contribute to "experiential avoidance." Thus, both processes may be successful in avoiding certain distressing experiences in the short term, yet contribute to their own problems and prevent the resolution of their key problems in the long term. Another way that (hypo)mania and depression are related is in the sense in which one is often a reaction to the other—driving mood upward to escape depression or suppressing activity to prevent a manic relapse.

We have encountered several metaphors that refer to this linking of high and low moods. A simple example is the idea that one "digs a deep hole" for oneself during depression, but "springs out" of the hole uncontrollably during a high. In another example, the following vignette illustrates how a female client begins a metaphor that the therapist grasps, and he suggests a possible way to build upon it:

Client: Well I put up this barrier against people so that they don't really know me. My husband doesn't like it at all. It's like a brick wall. The biggest barrier is when I am depressed and I completely withdraw from people.

Therapist: So is this brick wall always there, to some extent?

Client: No. When I am with my husband, I drop the barrier, but then I just start to worry about not being the perfect mother, the perfect wife, the perfect everything, so I try really hard to make him like me.

Therapist: So, you have this barrier that you drop with your husband. What is the trying to be perfect if it's not the barrier?

Client: Well it's like the barrier is down here [indicates] and then up here [indicates] it's like "I can doing anything, be perfect and hype myself up to be full of energy"

Therapist: So what is that then? Is it something you want to do?

Client: No, both of these are crap. They make things worse. They are both ways to protect myself, to not really be myself.

Therapist: It sounds to me like you are facing people like it's a war. You have this barrier down here to protect yourself [indicates], and then you have your weapons up here [indicates] which are your energy and you hyping yourself up.

Client: Yes, that's it! I have never really stopped protecting myself, except with you, because you don't have an agenda like everyone else.

Therapist: So what would happen if you dropped this barrier and put these weapons away in another situation?

Client: I don't know. I have never done it. Actually, yes I have. I have been putting my ideas "on the train" like you mentioned before.

Therapist: What's happening there?

Client: Well they are going round, and I don't have to act on them. Some of them don't even get on the train in the first place!

Therapist: So, it seems to be working?

Client: Yes, it really is.

Therapist: So, is there a situation where you might try out dropping your weapons and putting down the barrier?

Client: Yes, tonight, when my husband comes home. I could try not rushing around and trying to get the whole house perfect for when he comes back, and just see what happens.

In this dialogue, there are several metaphors. At the heart is a metaphor for the twin protective strategies of putting up an emotional barrier during depression and brandishing weapons during high-energy states. Both appear motivated by trying to avoid being seen as "not perfect" in other peoples' eyes. In earlier sessions it was apparent that this feared self-image involved feeling ridiculed and rejected by others, in a similar way to how she perceived that she had been rejected by her own father as a young child. The therapist attempted to work with the client in her generation and modification of the metaphor, checking in regularly to look for the client's additions and to check if his own suggestions seemed to fit. In this particular dialogue, the metaphor was used to ease the client into considering a behavioural experiment, but this is clearly not the core purpose of the metaphor; it is to help the client understand and shift perspectives on her presenting problem.

Another metaphor that we have encountered both within and outside the context of bipolar disorder, is the *boat on a rough sea*. The waves of the sea are a common metaphor for mood. Considering our evolutionary heritage, they may even form a universal symbol for mood, in a way not to dissimilar to Jung's idea of archetypes (Jung, 1964). Regardless of their origin, the image can be explored in a creative way within CBT. Clients often come to therapy feeling out of control of their mood, with the feeling that their mood controls them, rather than the other way round. The analogy of a boat, lost in a stormy sea, captures this felt sense. In this precarious situation, the person in the boat could not control the sea even if they tried—the sea is a natural force beyond human control. However, one can learn to manage, despite the sea—by anticipating the waves and directing the boat towards them to avoid capsizing. One can also build a stronger boat for future voyages and provide it with more effective means of steering its own path—sturdy sails or an outboard motor.

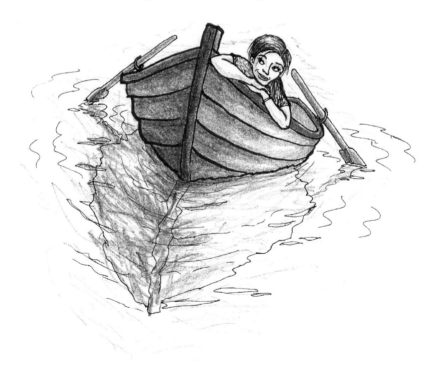

In a similar vein, people with bipolar disorder often need to accept that their moods are not easily controlled. Nevertheless, they can begin to reach their goals in life despite their mood through being aware of their own strengths and building upon them. When a sophisticated ocean liner is built to traverse the ocean, the waves rarely affect it, and it heads to its destination. This is not to deny that the weather at sea can be problematic. Nevertheless, by attending to the shipping forecast, particularly troublesome storms can be avoided. Similarly, people who recover from bipolar disorder, while they now tolerate a wider range of moods, are still very often aware of their limitations and may make prudent decisions at that time to avoid certain situations (e.g. challenging night shifts; working in the entertainment industry) without having a major impact on their quality of life in the long term.

Not only do people see their internal states in conflicting ways that seem to flip them from one phase to another. There are a cluster of related metaphors that highlight the conflicting beliefs about the whole condition of "bipolar disorder." One of these is the idea of bipolar disorder as a "dangerous gift"—a proclivity to be highly creative and productive that is also a source of danger than needs to be used wisely. One client described it as a gift that she would gladly return to the customer service counter of life! Yet other people have concluded the reverse—they would keep the "disorder," despite its dangers, because they believe that it is also the source of their talents and their positive experiences. Indeed, in the BBC2 documentary, *The Secret Life of the Manic Depressive* (2006), many people with bipolar disorder expressed this view. Stephen Fry, the interviewer, provided them with a metaphorical button that they could use to take away their bipolar disorder, both the highs and the lows. He placed it on the table in front of them, and only one of his interviewees chose to press it. The view that great talent and mental illness are entwined seems prevalent among sufferers, as well as the general public, and it is exemplified by the lives of highly successful individuals such as Vincent Van Gogh. In this way, iconic figures may serve as metaphors for a person's own experience of the inevitability of success and despair that characterizes the course of bipolar disorder.

Yet, if as health professionals, we are to help people with these perplexing and disabling conditions, we may need to step beyond this metaphor and examine it clearly. It is a patent fact that people can be creative without having a mental illness. Moreover it appears that people can have hypomanic experiences, and even hypomanic episodes, without developing bipolar disorder or needing treatment for a mental health problem (Seal, Mansell, & Mannion, 2008). Therefore, while our clients may need to give up some aspects of their highs, they may still be able to maintain much of their positive experiences and creativity during their recovery. They could be said to be "having their cake and eating it" rather than having it taken away by force and replaced with a rancid bun every time they visit the bakers!

The story of Icarus

The ancient Greek myth of Icarus can provide a richer way to explore the "dangerous gift" metaphor, both for clients and therapists. Many people are aware of the central message of this story—Icarus was able to fly yet he flew too close to the sun and burned his wings, tumbling to his death. In this respect, flight is the "dangerous gift." However, even in the first instance, this metaphor does not say that Icarus's crash was an inevitable consequence of his flying; he flew *too* close to the sun. What is *too* close? For a person with hypomanic experiences, their feelings of highs can have clear advantages to them, and during therapy these advantages are explored, in addition to considering when the risks and dangers may outweigh them. During CBT, clients can begin to consider what kinds of experiences are "too" high, and therefore require some kind of regulating strategy, and which ones may be acceptable.

The Icarus metaphor is wonderfully elaborate. In the myth, Icarus is the son of Daedalus, who was the creator of the infamous labyrinth in Crete that was commissioned by King Minos. The hero Theseus, another key figure of Greek mythology, was trapped within the labyrinth, which contained a Minotaur, a beast that was half-bull and half-man. Theseus was desperate to escape, and Daedalus, considerate of Theseus's plight, provided him with a route to escape. King Minos was so angry with his architect, that he locked Daedalus and Icarus in the labyrinth. Icarus was merely a child at the time, and so was condemned, through no fault of his own, to live his adolescent years in this dark, water-locked, subterranean maze, which paradoxically was his father's own creation. After many years, Daedalus used his gift of creativity to fashion Icarus wings so that he cold escape to freedom over the sea. According to the legend, he even explained to Icarus how to fly—keep above the sea so that the feathers do not get wet—and below the sun so that they do not burn. However, when Icarus set forth, he became enraptured by the warmth of a sun that he had not felt or seen since his early years, and his father's warnings became realized—he crashed to the sea and drowned.

Rather than point out every point of reference within the Icarus metaphor, we have provided some key examples in Table 8.2. Within this book, we have generally been describing simple metaphors that fit relatively easily into Socratic, client-centred CBT. The Icarus story is clearly of a different kind, and comparable to the way that other myths, fables, and even novels, movies and biographies can be used as metaphors for a client's predicament. They can

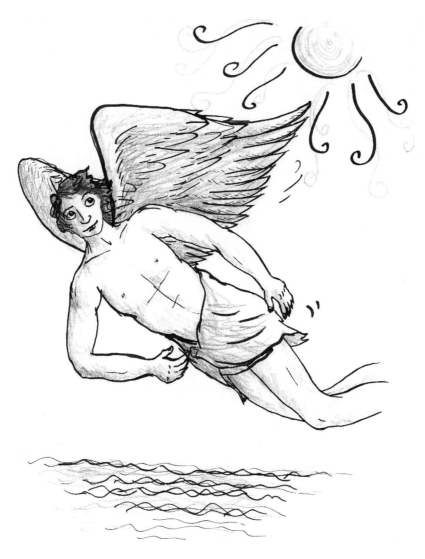

potentially provide a longitudinal, narrative conceptualization that is lacking in brief metaphors. The Icarus metaphor itself has been used in training about CBT for bipolar disorder to health professionals, in order to try to dispel simple explanations of mood episodes, and to provide a visual metaphor for a developmental and psychological conceptualization of the disorder. It also engenders sympathy for individuals, whose behaviour can be frustrating for others and be seen as a deliberate attempt to increase risk. We can also imagine that it could be used in group CBT for bipolar disorder, where the disclosure of personal accounts may initially prove too sensitive to discuss.

Table 8.2 Examples of key facets of the story of Icarus and their potential links with the experience and history of an individual with bipolar disorder

Metaphor component	Feature of bipolar disorder
Icarus is imprisoned for his youth in a labyrinth	Confusion; feeling lost; aversive childhood experiences
The cause of imprisonment is unjust (Daedelus and Icarus were both punished for Daedelus helping Theseus to escape)	Feelings of injustice and resentment over past childhood experiences (e.g. Mansell & Hodson, 2008)
Wings provide an escape from the labyrinth	Using high mood and energy states to rise above adversity; sometimes called a "manic defence"
Daedelus made the wings for Icarus	Parent provides the influential model of high creativity and productivity
Daedelus gives Icarus advice on how to fly between the sun and sea	Advice provided by family and health professionals, that is often ignored
Warmth of the sun attracts Icarus	The high feelings are seductive and overcome advice or reason, especially when contrasted with past adversity and negative feelings
The sun burns Icarus's wings and he tumbles to his death	The highs can end in catastrophe if pushed to an extreme
Icarus needed to fly above the sea so as not get his wings wet, and below the sun so as not to burn them	The idea of maintaining a "safe bandwidth" of mood—a potential recovery strategy that permits some highs and lows

Recovery

Across a range of mental health problems, recovery is associated with greater self-acceptance and understanding. Having experienced the chaotic ups and downs of bipolar disorder, recovery often seems to involve some acceptance of one's limitations and a choice to live within the bounds of experience that are shared with other people. These quotes—provided by a client who worked with a colleague of ours, Sarah Goff—illustrate this process using metaphor:

> I have begun to realise that manic depression is just as much part of me as my size 8 feet, my brown eyes, my eye for words. And once you realise it is part of your being, then you act accordingly. I respect my size 8 feet by giving them size 8 shoes to live in; otherwise I would be crippled. But once I have bought my shoes I do not give the size my feet are labelled another thought. Similarly I try to respect my manic depression by taking my medication, by eating properly, by sleeping (or at least resting) at a conventional time. Otherwise I am often emotionally and physically drained. I've given up resenting manic depression; sometimes I feel glad I have it.

A second quote illustrates self-acceptance combined with a metaphor for the oscillating highs and lows, and the acceptable middle ground in between:

> I feel as I have finally learnt what it is like to walk along the pavement with the rest of humanity, rather than to be either digging around in a pothole (depression) or scrambling up a lamp-post (hypomania/mania). Being stuck with just dank brown mud in a pothole has no appeal, and while the view from a lamp-post was often quite spectacular (being wider than that of those who meandered along the pavement) it was not the most comfortable place to perch, and it hurt when one fell off! (often into another pothole). But a pavement—indeed it is initially uninspiring, being flat and well trodden—but one can wander anywhere on a pavement, admire all sorts of wonderful things, meet all sorts of people, and yet remain in a safe, stable environment. I have discovered the joys of living with the throng on the pavement…walking on the pavement has freed my mind from expending energy on clambering out of holes or down from lamp-posts, and I can use this energy more productively. Above all, now that this condition is recognized and held at bay, I am learning to trust my mind – therefore to trust myself. And thus to like being me.

Another key theme in recovery from bipolar disorder seems to be the assertion of autonomy. Until then, many of our clients report that they feel driven to push themselves and succeed not for themselves, but to prove themselves to others. They seem driven to suppress recurrent childhood memories of being seen as a failure, or "never good enough" by parents, teachers and other role models by extreme goal-striving (Mansell & Hodson, 2009; Mansell & Lam, 2004). In many ways, the drive to hypo(mania) can be fueled by an attempt to challenge these expectations, but they fail to do so because of the chaotic effects on thinking and behaviour that are associated with states of high mood that lead to more problems, and then greater dependency. During recovery they report that they learn how to assert their own needs and to successfully challenge other people's evaluations of them rather than conform with them. There are many metaphors from movies that capture this process—from the sublime to the ridiculous: there is the beguiling way that the protagonist in *Strictly Ballroom* confounds the critics of his innovative dancing routine, to the humourous way that the young chef in *Ratatouille* confronts the conspiracy and ridicule he experiences from his fellow chefs after he commits to intensive training with a creative rat that inhabits his chef's hat and guides his every move. Probably the most pertinent example is *Shine*, which tells the true story of a musician Peter Helfgott who had been "diagnosed" with various conditions at different times, including bipolar disorder. The movie illustrates the early punitive social pressures to perform that he experiences during childhood, the catastrophic effects on his mental health during adulthood, and his eventual recovery as he forms an unconditional positive relationship with a partner who meets him at his worst and helps him to reclaim his life.

Recovery metaphors can be useful not only to the client generating them during the process itself, but they can also act as an inspiration for people who are more troubled by their mood swings at present. Within therapy groups, clients often share their difficult experiences and how they coped with them. On a larger scale, sharing metaphors of recovery provides a potentially stronger theme of how coping is achieved at an attitudinal level. We are yet to see how metaphors like the ones quoted here can impact on recovery groups for bipolar disorder, but we would expect them to be particularly helpful.

Summary

In this chapter, we have illustrated how clients' own metaphors of their internal states—mood, arousal, cognition, and behaviour—are particularly fruitful to identify and explore as they help to unpack their experiences, and the often extreme and conflicting appraisals of these states. Metaphors can help clients to view their highs and lows as ways of coping with other longstanding problems such as feelings of failure or past trauma. Through taking a recovery perspective, we can utilize stories, either real or fictional, to help clients to see their experiences in perspective and head towards a future self (or selves) that is more resilient and yet still feels genuine to the client—the "real me."

Chapter 9

Psychosis

Introduction

Arguably, psychosis represents the paradigm example of extreme psychological distress. People who have experienced psychosis report a combination of unusual perceptual phenomena, bizarre thoughts and beliefs, extreme emotions, and feelings of confusion, and loss of control. Some of the "classic" psychotic symptoms include auditory hallucinations (hearing voices), delusions (beliefs that are deemed unacceptable or bizarre by one's surrounding culture), and thought disorder (tangential thinking and associations; difficulties maintaining thoughts on a fixed topic). Psychosis characterizes the "psychotic disorders," such as schizophrenia, schizoaffective disorder, and delusional disorder. These are deemed to be serious mental illnesses because of the major impact on life and relationships that these experiences typically have for people who are diagnosed with these disorders. In addition, psychosis can be experienced by people with other diagnoses, such as borderline personality disorder, major depression, and bipolar disorder. Given the uniqueness of this state, its widespread relevance, and its potential destructiveness, it is important for us as clinicians to consider better ways to understand and empathize with the experience.

In reviewing the literature on metaphors and psychosis, we found that the relationship between psychosis and metaphor was broader than we had imagined. Specifically, we discovered four different relationships between the two. They are the following:

1. *Psychosis as a metaphor.* For example, the term "schizophrenic" has been used metaphorically in the media to describe two incompatible views on a topic (e.g. "a schizophrenic approach to policy making")

2. *Prevalent metaphors.* Metaphors that are commonly used, either explicitly or implicitly, to try to explain psychosis.

3. *Metaphorical processing during psychosis.* Many accounts of psychosis have identified that the psychotic state involves substantial use of metaphor.

4. *Metaphors that are helpful for people with psychosis.* Many of these are reported by therapists and others within genuine or fictional accounts of recovery.

The last point clearly describes the category we are most interested in for the purposes of the book, but the first three also deserve some attention and so we will cover these before introducing metaphors in CBT directly.

Psychosis as a metaphor

The use of psychosis itself as a metaphor is rarely a helpful enterprise, least of all for the individuals with that label. The term "schizophrenic" has developed its own meaning relating to being in two minds, based on an inaccurate lay belief that schizophrenia is characterized by twin personalities. Critically, the term "schizophrenic" is nearly always used in a pejorative sense, as though having two opinions on a topic is close to mental instability. We do not have any more to say about this phenomenon except that where clients or their families raise this area of confusion themselves, the therapist can listen to and validate any distress caused, and go some way to attempt to clarify the term. The therapist may help also redirect the client to their own opinions. What does the label mean to the client, independently of what others believe?

Prevalent metaphors

The most prevalent metaphors for psychosis are often limited, and sometimes counterproductive. Psychosis, or more often schizophrenia, is often directly regarded as an illness, or metaphorically compared to a physical illness such as diabetes or heart disease. The parallels are obvious—there are physical changes associated with acute episodes and they often entail medication or going into hospital. The advantage of viewing psychosis as an illness may include that the individual appreciates that they have a significant problem, and that they seek help when they can no longer cope by themselves. The disadvantages include a view that medication is always necessary, that the condition is life-long (like diabetes), and that psychological interventions cannot help.

It can be very helpful to discuss the mental model that clients have of their psychosis, just as in other psychological problems (see Chapter 4, p. 70). We believe that it is important for the therapist to listen closely to the client's model, accept this as the client's own starting point, and yet explore alternative models that the client may sometimes entertain, or be able to develop. The aim is not to directly contradict a medical model straight away, but to examine its validity for the client in question. There is also the issue of *which* medical model and, moreover, their level of knowledge about the illness they are using as an analogy. For example, the client may describe their psychosis as like a cancer, which to them is completely outside their control, aggressive, and fated to end in disaster. The therapist can discuss whether cancer is always like this—how do we account for people who recover from cancer? If it is possible to think of cancer differently, is another metaphor more appropriate, or could the client recover from psychosis too under certain circumstances? A further possibility for clients who closely adhere to a medical model is that a helpful, sophisticated and flexible metaphor for psychosis can be introduced that is nevertheless partly based on a medical model. We introduce this later in the context of the "synesthesia metaphor" for voices.

Another metaphor often used relates to the stress-vulnerability model—it is like having a *bucket with a hole* in it at the side—as the bucket fills up with

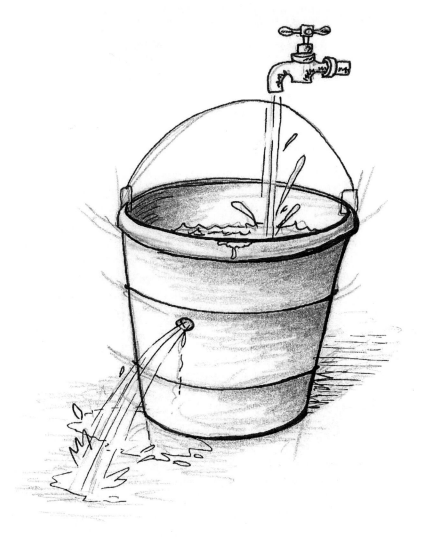

water there is a greater and greater chance it will leak. In this metaphor, the water is the stress and the bucket with a hole in is the vulnerable individual. A similar metaphor involves a pressure cooker under a stove that is gradually increasing in temperature until it bursts. These metaphors potentially enforce the notion both that the client is "vulnerable" and that the way of coping is to reduce the amount of "stress" in their lives. This may help individuals who would otherwise not acknowledge their vulnerability, or who might have previously regarded such vulnerability as fixed and independent of stress. But this conceptualization has drawbacks. What is the client to define as "stress"? How do we know whether they are making choices that enable them to cope or ones that limit their life unnecessarily? These metaphors can be adapted to assist the client. For example the skills that the client learns, including cognitive reappraisal, can be visualized as making the bucket larger—providing more space and therefore less likelihood of overflow. While this metaphor may have its uses at certain stages, for example in a focused relapse prevention module, it seems rather static to us, with little versatility to consider the multifaceted experiences of psychosis and recovery.

Metaphorical processing during psychosis

The relationship between the psychotic state and metaphor has been apparent for a long time. Here is one example from one of our own clients. "Harry" was a 23-year-old man whose first psychotic episode involved the delusion that his face had been disfigured when his "friends" at university mixed poison with his drink in a party. He became extremely paranoid that they would do it again and turn him "ugly." During therapy, he revealed that when he was a child at school, he had once fallen asleep in class and his friends had shaved one of his eyebrows off as a "joke." It appeared that Harry's psychotic experiences were a metaphor for an actual experience that had continued to upset him with a feeling of betrayal and social rejection. Harry and his family found it very helpful to realise that his beliefs were not "mad" and incomprehensible, but reflected the themes of an earlier aversive experience. This kind of linkage in psychotic clients has been observed over the years, originally within a psychodynamic approach:

> Actually the only thing "wrong" as it were with the so-called "schizophrenic" is that he speaks in metaphors unacceptable to his audience, particularly his psychiatrist.

> (Thomas Szasz, 1976, p. 14)

> Communication is of the essence, and the client is often weaned from his autistic preoccupations and his idiosyncratic communications by the therapist's ability to hear and understand what the client wishes to say even while he seeks to conceal through the use of idiosyncratic metaphor and cryptic associations.

> (Theodore Lidz, 1973. p 10, 103)

It is not surprising that the best writing about psychosis, and particularly schizo-phrenia, depends so heavily on metaphor. Psychosis is, after all, a sort of over-extended metaphor, an ultimately unsuccessful but nevertheless creative attempt to impose a comprehensible pattern on the universe.

(Eve Zibart, 2008; Interview with Lauren Slater)

Perhaps the most intriguing account of recent years has been provided by Joe Griffin and Ivan Tyrell (2006). They review a range of clinical, cognitive, and neurophysiological evidence to conclude that psychosis is characterized by "waking reality processed through a dreaming brain." They note that the REM state is characterized by metaphors as reported within accounts of dreaming, and that there are striking similarities between the style of processing in dreams and the accounts of people with psychosis. They recognize that clients who have experienced psychosis often report that it had felt as though they had been trapped in a dreaming state. Their recommended intervention involves asking the client about their metaphors during psychosis and working with them to help modify their meanings. This is designed to help them understand what they are going through and make choices about whether to spend more time in waking reality. This approach shares common ground with the cogni-tive approach adopted in this book. Griffin and Tyrell (2006) go on to propose that the ability for people to "dream while awake" is very functional and is at the root of our ability to be creative and imaginative. There are parallels here between this theory and those that we covered in Chapter 2 (p. 17)—meta-phors and dreams capture the capacity for sensorimotor simulation of poten-tial experiences and courses of action to allow potential problems to be resolved within an imagining mode of cognition. However, exactly how we are to dis-tinguish between dreaming, psychosis, the creative use of metaphor, and other forms of planning and simulation is yet to be operationalized. This is critical however, as they clearly vary widely in their level of functionality.

We have some sympathy for the linkage between psychosis and metaphori-cal thought for several reasons. First, while the cognitive and behavioural maintenance mechanisms in psychosis are relatively well understood (e.g. Garety et al., 2001; Morrison, 2001), the explanation for the phenomenology of the psychotic state is much less clear and there appears to be little consensus within the psychological literature. Therefore, any scientific account that pur-ports to fill this gap is worth considering, including that of Griffin and Tyrell. Second, cognitive formulation of psychosis proposes that schematic links do indeed exist between the metaphors provided by clients and the nature of their interpersonal and intrapersonal problems. Perhaps the most striking example of this is reported in a detailed paper on imagery in psychosis by Tony Morrison and colleagues (Morrison et al., 2002). Morrison and colleagues found links between the content of intrusive imagery and past traumas of their

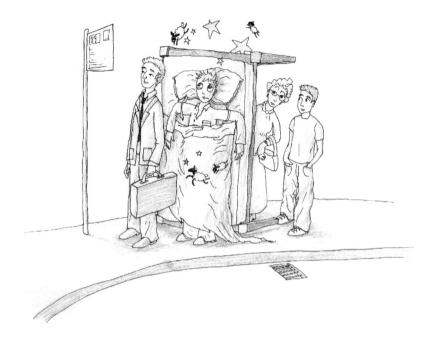

participants—for some this was a direct nonmetaphorical connection (e.g. image of self rocking in a psychiatric hospital); for others, the connection was metaphorical (e.g. an image of being chopped up by axes related to an experience of being physically assaulted in a pub).

Our third reason for utilizing this literature is that our own experience indicates that clients find it useful to relate psychotic experiences to dreaming for several reasons. A dream is a real experience that happens to everyone and can have a huge emotional impact on them (e.g. during a nightmare). Yet, we do not hold people accountable for what they do in a dream, nor do we expect a dream to be a direct reflection of reality. Thus, this metaphor has the capacity to normalize the experience of psychosis while validating its capacity to induce distress, despite it not necessarily reflecting the reality of the real-life situation. The collaborative discussion of similarities and difference between psychosis and dreaming (or nightmares) can be a very fruitful way to explore meaning with clients and help them to gain a sense of control and acceptance of the experience. In a published article, J. M. Tolton (2006), who recovered from psychosis, summed it up in the following way:

> If a delusion is only a waking nightmare and not reality, then what is there to worry about? (p. 488)

Metaphors in CBT for psychosis

In this section, we cover three classes of metaphor used in CBT for psychosis: metacognitive, interpersonal, and narrative.

Metacognitive approaches to delusional thinking

There are a diverse range of experiences that come under the umbrella of psychosis. In this section, we focus on two key domains—"delusional" thoughts and voices—and explore how to help clients take a helpful metacognitive stance towards them.

The metacognitive approach helps to intersect the idea of a delusion. If a person with psychosis can detect the thoughts that have delusional themes as soon as they arise in awareness, this gives them the opportunity to catch and reflect on them, rather than accepting them as fact. Freeman & Garety (2004) evoked a metaphor from the writing of Francis Bacon to bring this idea to life:

> Suspicions amongst thoughts are like bats amongst birds—they ever fly by twilight. Certainly they are to be repressed, or, at the least, well guarded. For they cloud the mind, they lose friends, and they check with business, whereby business cannot go on currently and constantly. They dispose kings to tyranny, husbands to jealousy, wise men to irresolution and melancholy.

(Francis Bacon (1625) cited in Freeman & Garety, 2004)

Andrew Gumley and Matthias Schwannhauer have illustrated how paranoid thoughts can build up into a fully fledged belief in a steady drip-by-drip process. During training for CBT, they use a clip from *Lord of the Rings: Return of the King* where Gollum is whispering comments to Frodo that suggest to him that his friend, Sam, is plotting to steal the prized ring. Each comment is based on evidence that Frodo can see with his own eyes, but each is provided a paranoid interpretation by Gollum. The circumstances of this process are important to and appear analogous to those experienced in the lead up to psychosis—there is a context of danger provided by the perilous journey they are taking up a dark rocky mountain path, the physical strain and limited sleep involved, and then a single "solution" to the potential catastrophe in the form of the golden ring. Eventually this accumulation of stress and apparent evidence tips the balance, and Frodo abandons his friend. There are parallels here in the features of stories that clients provide, especially in the early stages of psychosis. The *Lord of the Rings* sequence can provide a discussion tool for training and a primer for identifying these kinds of encroaching factors in the development of paranoia.

A somewhat similar process has been described by J. M. Tolton, mentioned earlier. After recovery, he built a theory of how his delusional thinking had developed, which he termed a "rogue psychotic mindset," which he viewed as analogous to stored information about other topics:

> It occurred to me that the large group of misconceived ideas, beliefs and thoughts could be regarded as a set of information in the same way as, for example, mathematics or English literature. The difference being that my academic knowledge is largely factual, whereas, my rogue psychotic mindset is full of fictional delusive nonsense. Examples of what I perhaps loosely define as mindsets are language, science, social skills, criminal intent, politics and economics, music, work skills, computer skills and sport skills. At the point where I went psychotic, I was desperately searching my mind for an explanation as to what was happening to me. I was drawing on mindsets such as C.S.E. physics to provide the reason for this new and terrifying psychotic state of mind and body. I was now mentally clutching at straws.

> I began to fill the factual information void with misconceived ideas that were baseless and cobbled together from incomplete, weak and unsuitable mindsets. For me it was like having a life skills manual, which is suddenly found to have certain critical sections missing. Recovery from serious mental illness ultimately requires the gaps to be soundly filled in.

> The delusion may remain in memory but takes the form of a frozen memory fossil rather than a rogue cognition that can drive a sufferer into inappropriate behaviour.

In this account, Tolton clearly extends the metaphor further, regarding the development of a psychotic explanation as analogous to "cobbling together" explanations when the critical pages are missing from a "life skills manual." As mentioned in Chapter 5, to aid his recovery, Tolton had developed a process of checking his thoughts as they appeared for their "delusive content" and used a poem (reproduced in Chapter 5, p. 100) to prompt him to do this. The metaphor he uses to describe his psychotic mindset after recovery is interesting too—a "memory fossil," which presumably no longer maintains the living capacity to incorporate itself into his explanations as in the past.

It can be helpful to take a metacognitive approach with clients who report unusual beliefs, even if they may seem to be held with a strong conviction. In Chapter 5, we covered a range of analogies that can be used to help examine thoughts when clients find it difficult to grasp the metacognitive approach. For example, the metaphor of watching leaves on a river, or carriages of a train, passing by can help to provide the kind of decentred approach that may help them to manage their lives despite the intrusions that they experience. In some of our work with people who have delusional beliefs, it can be greatly empowering simply to delineate an intrusive thought that reflects the delusion from a fully held delusional belief that can determine behaviour and impact on functioning. This can remove the stigma and perceived catastrophe from delusional thoughts and provide the individual with a chance to consider more helpful perspectives on their situation.

Metacognitive approaches to hearing voices

It must be difficult for anyone who has not heard voices to appreciate the nature of the voice-hearing experience. Voice-hearers typically describe their voice as a real entity with which they have a good, bad, or mixed relationship. They often explain that their voices are as loud, or louder, than people talking in their environment, and this is often apparent from their distractibility during conversation as their attention is caught by them.

It can be very helpful to use metaphors to explain the experience of voice hearing to family members, health professionals, and therapists, thereby promoting empathy and understanding of the clients. We have encountered several examples. Andrew Gumley and Matthias Schwannhauer use a sequence from the *Lord of the Rings: The Two Towers*, where one character is in dialogue with himself: Smeagol is the name given to his caring side, whereas Gollum is the name given to the manipulative side who dominated the individual's mind after corruption by the powerful ring that forms the focus of the story.

Ian Lowens provided us with another analogy familiar to psychologists who have studied selective attention—the "cocktail party" effect (see also Chapter 7, p. 132). In a busy cocktail party full of chatty guests it is difficult to focus one's attention on one person's voice and ignore the others. This is made particularly difficult if other people are gossiping about "hot" topics—the emotional salience of their conversation captures your attention. In the same way, voices compete for attention with speech from people in the outside environment, and their content is often more emotionally salient whether praising, criticizing, or commanding the person experiencing them. This metaphor can be used both to validate and explain the difficulties in concentration and engagement with others that voice-hearers can experience, in addition to providing clinicians with an illustrative example of the voice-hearing experience. A further method, commonly used in training, is for pairs to role-play a conversation with a third person talking into the ear of one of the pair. The interference effect of the voice is soon apparent.

In the remaining part of this section, we provide an illustration of how a specific metaphor has been used to work with voice hearing based on the analogy with a condition known as synesthesia. People with this condition (or skill) merge their sensory modalities in a way that most of us would find bizarre; they report that they can hear colours or see sounds, for example.

In this specific example, Aidan Bucknall worked with a client who was socially isolated and heard voices that were for the most part benign and to a

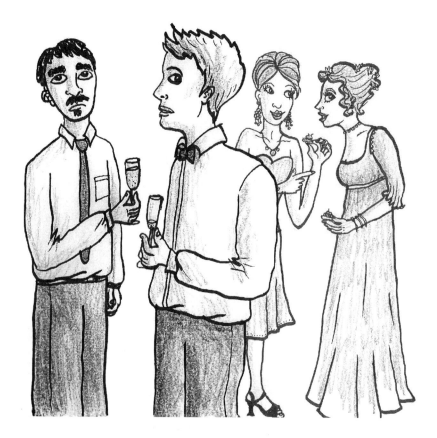

certain extent kept the client occupied and provided him with company. Yet, occasionally the voices would be very critical and aversive. In discussing the voices with the client, the therapist was trying to formulate a different way of understanding the voices because even the benign voices fundamentally disturbed him. The client came from an affluent family who found it hard to accept and cope with the idea of a mental illness and the stigma that it implies. The client himself regarded the voices as an illness, which in turn he stigmatized, indicating that he was "the lowest of the low" in society. Nevertheless, the voices appeared to provide an experience of mundane social contact in the absence of a social life in his environment.

The therapist struggled to find a mental model of the voices that provided an alternative to the medical approach the client reported. In this instance, the therapist had been reading about synesthesia, and he introduced this condition to the client. He asked the client whether he had heard of synesthesia. The client had not, but was keen to read up about it for homework. In this instance, synesthesia provided a suitable metaphor for the client's experiences. They worked on the ideas that psychosis was like synesthesia: internal events (imagination) triggered a very different sensory experience (voices). It proved to be a handy neuropsychological metaphor to work with, that seemed to fit with the client's medical slant on his problem.

The metaphor also helped the therapist to empathize with the client's predicament. Imagine if you were to actually hear your thoughts as voices, then they would be almost as real to you as someone sitting in the room with you and you might begin to build your whole life around them. The client went on to use this idea to explain his voices to other people: "It's like my imagination in sound form," thereby being both medically grounded and yet at the same time providing other people with an idea of his experience and reducing potential stigmatization. Thus, he felt more confident to talk to other people. A further metaphor was introduced at this later stage to describe the process whereby the client took control of his own explanation of his experiences; he became the "script writer," and given that he is the writer, he could now choose the genre of script—a recovery story rather than a tragedy. This role is itself empowering and helped him to rise above seeing himself as the victim of the voices. We will return to the narrative function of metaphors in the recovery from psychosis later in the chapter.

Interpersonal processes

The social impact of psychosis is huge. Part of this can relate to the sheer fear of attack or persecution that many sufferers experience in the company of other people. The client is often hypervigilant for threats from other people, jumps to conclusions about their malevolent intentions, and may employ a range of safety behaviours such as reduced eye contact, avoidance of situations, and worry. Therefore it is often helpful to work on understanding anxiety and how it affects attention, reasoning, and safety behaviours in a similar way to anxiety disorders. We covered metaphors on this topic in detail in Chapter 7.

An immediate impact of a client's fear of others is on the therapeutic relationship, often limiting the kinds of questioning or techniques that can be used. For example, Ian Lowens has shared with us how he manages with clients who find it threatening to be asked Socratic questions about their experiences. In these clients, the question, "What do these thoughts mean to you?" can be felt as undermining because they can imply that the client must be mistaken, and therefore stupid for thinking this way. In contrast, a more visual and collaborative path is ensured through an alternative approach. Ian asks them whether they have a picture of what is happening to them right now. What is in this picture? What could I see if I was looking at this with you? This style of questioning, which uses a picture or a painting as a metaphor for their thoughts or feelings, makes it clearer that the questions are not designed to be a test, but to aid a joint understanding, in the spirit of CBT.

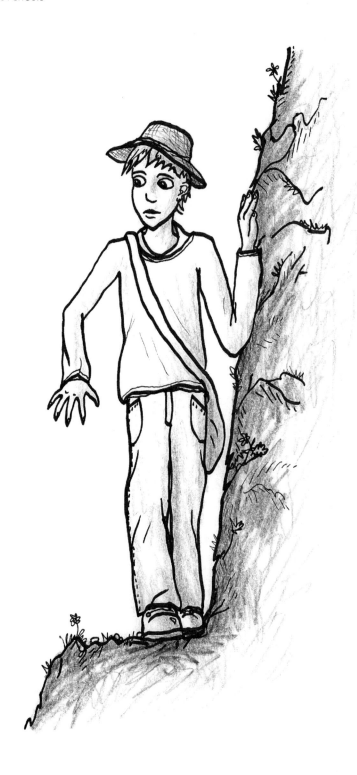

The suspicious thoughts of a person with psychosis often reflect a broader fear of connecting with other people. A key dilemma our clients experience is whether to risk engaging with other people who might harm or reject them, or to continue to avoid other people and lose the opportunity to live a fulfilling life with them. Ian Lowens sometimes uses a metaphor of a narrow path with a vast drop on one side to represent this dilemma for his clients. This metaphor is particularly versatile in how it can be explored. For example, the sheer effort and concentration that would be needed to traverse this narrow path becomes evident to both therapist and client and helps to validate the stress that the client experiences. The therapist can also work with the width of this path—how narrow is it? Is it narrow for the whole length (i.e. in every situation) Whereabouts might it be wider? Would you risk stepping more to the side and letting go of your usual effort to remain as far from the edges as possible? These elaborations of the metaphor provide possible entry points to behavioural experiments about testing out contact with other people, starting with the safest situations first. The metaphor can even be extended more creatively—is there space on the path for me? (i.e. can the therapist be trusted in some circumstances?); can you see what is at the end of the pathway? (i.e. could you share with me the goal that might motivate you to face some difficult social situations?) This metaphor is clearly one that can be used in other client groups where they describe a regular dilemma of weighing up what appear to be two very threatening courses of action during their lives.

Narratives of psychosis in popular culture

There are many richly descriptive narratives of psychosis and the recovery process that can provide validation and encouragement for service users. In a literary angle on this topic, Wolfe and Wolfe (1976) pointed to the similarities between these accounts. They noted that the titles of many of these accounts reflect a metaphor that sets the tone for the entire work: *The Snake Pit; The Prison of My Mind; Labyrinth of Silence; Halfway Through the Tunnel; The Invisible Curtain; The Bell Jar.* The common theme here is that psychosis is a state of feeling trapped in a confusing, dark, subterranean, and threatening place. In contrast, the story of recovery in many of these accounts reflects an emergence from disorder to order, during an ascent into an ordered environment. In one of these accounts, *I Never Promised You a Rose Garden* by Joanne Greenberg, the story of recovery was reflected by the imagery of mountains. The journey up the mountain represented to struggle to reclaim mental stability and view the world for what it is at this higher level, rather than as a chaotic underworld. It is worth noting from what we covered in Chapter 8 that the experience of psychosis is likely to be somewhat different in people who have been psychotic following a high mood state, such as during mania. For them, even positive mood states can be associated with distressing psychotic experiences.

In addition to the bounty of books on the psychotic experience, the number of fictional and autobiographical films is impressive too (see Wedding, Boyd, & Niemec, 2005). We have found *Donnie Darko*, *A Beautiful Mind*, and *The Fisher King* to be particularly informative. Often, clients have already seen these films and so they provide an entry point to discuss the narrative perspective on psychosis.

Donnie Darko is richest in its use of metaphor. In this movie, Donnie is a teenager diagnosed with paranoid psychosis who hallucinates a man-sized skull-faced rabbit (an embodiment of ambivalence?) called Frank who instructs him to commit acts of destruction in the countdown to the end of the world. One of the key features of this movie is that its narrative is convoluted and ambiguous in meaning, thereby echoing the experience of psychosis. It also acutely critiques the helping profession in the form of a self-aggrandizing self-help guru, an emotionally naïve teacher, and an intrusive hypnotherapist. We have not yet used this movie in CBT but we imagine that it echoes the frustrations that people with psychosis experience at the hands of society and those who are meant to be able to understand their predicament.

A Beautiful Mind tells the true story of the talented mathematician John Nash, who developed schizophrenia for a long period of his life and now experiences a measured level of recovery. This movie illustrates the subjective nature of reality very well because the transition between "what actually happened" and the protagonist's delusional version of events is deliberately unclear, such that the viewer is drawn into John's perception. It also provides an empowering story of how someone with schizophrenia can achieve success and recover to some degree by managing with ongoing psychotic experiences. At the end of the film, he is still hearing voices, but he is more open about them to others and appears to take an active choice to attend and engage with people in his environment.

The Fisher King tells the story of a man who develops an eccentric form of psychosis after his wife is murdered in a random killing and falls into a life on the streets. Yet, through his evolving and mutually supportive companionship with a radio DJ, he begins to reclaim his life. Among other things, this film illustrates that psychosis can be triggered by traumatic events in contrast to a purely medical account. It also illustrates the importance of friendship and the hope of recovery.

Summary

Metaphor and psychosis are intrinsically linked within phenomenology, cognitive style, and the process of therapy. While there is little written specifically on the use of metaphor in psychotic clients, our overview would indicate that it is a fruitful avenue to pursue. Indeed, given the extent to which people in acute states appear to be consumed by a metaphorical form of processing, using metaphors may provide the most helpful bridge in meaning between the client and the therapist. Indeed, the constructive use of metaphor in CBT may illustrate the appropriate balance between analogical and analytical thinking that a person with a history of psychosis can strive for during their recovery. This area is clearly ripe for research, theory, and innovations in practice, which we anticipate with eagerness.

Chapter 10

Eating disorders

Introduction

Eating disorders refer to a complex, often dangerous and sometimes life-threatening group of problems, predominantly (but not exclusively) affecting women. Anorexic problems involve purposeful and persistent restriction of food intake such that body weight drops into a dangerously low range. Bulimic problems involve a repetitive cycle of excessive, uncontrolled binge eating followed by some form of compensatory behaviour such as intentional vomiting. Various cognitive behavioural approaches have been put forward to conceptualize and treat eating disorders (Wolff & Serpell, 1998; Waller et al., 2007; Fairburn, Shafran & Cooper, 1999; Fairburn, Cooper, & Shafran, 2003; Treasure & Schmidt, 2006). However, treatment outcomes are as yet modest, particularly for the anorexic population.

Working with clients with eating disorders can be an enormous challenge: individuals often value their disorder highly and find it difficult to conceptualize as a problem. Consequently, they may lack motivation to change and feel very ambivalent about engaging in treatment. Additionally, individuals with eating disorders tend to have a black-and-white thinking style, difficulties with cognitive flexibility, and a tendency to miss the bigger picture because of an overfocus on detail (Lopez et al., 2008). Idiosyncratic beliefs about the meaning and function of food and eating are often developed over time and become rigid and "stuck" as the client has increasing difficulty seeing outside the ever-smaller box her life has become. The use of metaphors in therapy may be of great use in working with clients who have an eating disorder for these and other reasons.

This chapter explores use of metaphor across several key areas within eating disorders work. It begins with a look at the "imprisoning" effect eating disorders often have upon clients, and how sufferers can feel "little" both psychologically and physically. The chapter will then consider metaphor use in addressing the meaning and function of food, and how to usefully consider eating disorders as an external entity. Finally, the chapter will consider the problems when self-evaluation becomes too narrowly defined in terms of eating, shape, and weight, and the issue of balancing psychological and medical needs in this population.

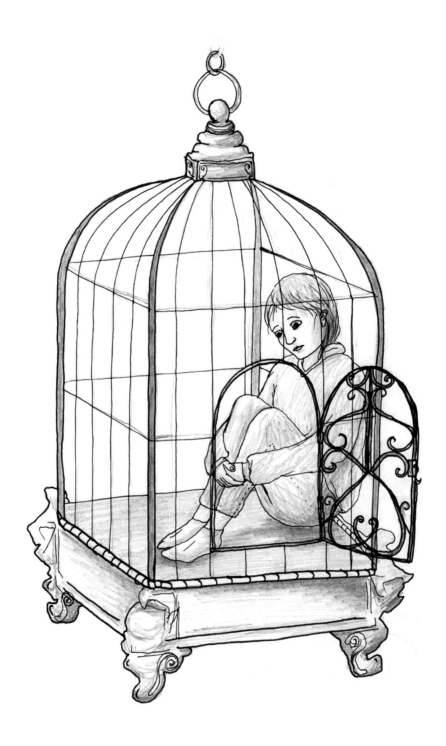

The gilded cage

This idea of being "imprisoned" or "caged in" by an eating disorder is a good place to start when considering the use of metaphors with this group. Many clients spontaneously describe their eating disorder as feeling "like a cage," and this can be developed in various ways. Is the cage gilded or does it have hard iron bars? If the door opened, would they try to escape? Or would they remain within the safe confines of their prison? The idea of the cage or prison can evoke powerful imagery, and some clients have found it meaningful and motivating to create drawings or other images around this theme. This metaphor is clearly not unique to eating disorders and can be applied to any long-term problem with which a client is highly ambivalent, such as bipolar disorder, obsessive-compulsive disorder, or an addiction.

Little lives, little selves

The experience and pursuit of "littleness" is common in eating disorder clients and has a fundamentally metaphorical nature to it. Eating disorder clients often report feeling their lives have got smaller or "shrunk" so that relationships, friends, family, work, and hobbies have all been lost or marginalized in favour of the eating disorder.

This contraction of life may be powerfully mirrored, particularly for anorexic clients, by an actual physical shrinking of the self. The small physical self of the anorexic client may take on various idiosyncratic metaphorical meanings, which can be useful to consider in therapy. One client had a mental image of herself as a tiny person, only a few inches high, surrounded by powerful others who towered over her. For this client, her increasingly small physical size had become a metaphor for how she perceived herself in relation to others. In a variation on this, another client described her perception of herself:

> I take up too much room, I'm just too much, I spill out everywhere. I want to vanish, to be so small that people don't notice me, to be little and neat and quiet.

For this client, her anorexia was a way to diminish and control a self she felt was uncontainable. Exploring how the physical self can become a metaphor for psychological states and processes may facilitate a new perspective on the function of her eating disorder for a client as well as providing valuable information for the formulation.

Food, eating, and weight gain

Clients with eating disorders often develop characteristic and strongly held beliefs about the meaning and function of food. Many clients lose sight of the idea of food as necessary for their bodies to function properly. The following two, "food as fuel" metaphors, contributed by Glenn Waller and his team at St George's Hospital can be useful to make this point. The first, "keeping the car going" is useful when discussing the importance of maintaining carbohydrate intake levels to provide energy in a balanced eating program rather than just eating vegetables or protein: "Imagine that you have a car. You put in the best oil there is. The brake fluid that you use is the most highly recommended on the market. Your screen wash wins awards. However, you do not put in any petrol. How would you expect the car to perform?"

The "filling up the car" metaphor can be used to try to encourage a client that she needs to eat adequate amounts at each meal and snack: "If you were to give your car one liter of petrol at a time, you would never be out of the 'red' zone in your car's fuel gauge. You spend all your time searching for the next filling station, and you are unlikely to enjoy the trip, because you are constantly anxious and can only think about where the next little bit of fuel is coming from."

Somewhat similar to these is the "food as medicine" metaphor. Clients often describe not being hungry, not liking food, or not liking the sort of food they need to eat to recover their health. In these situations, it can be useful to introduce this idea, as illustrated in the dialogue below:

Client: Well it got to 11am and I just wasn't hungry so I didn't eat my snack.
Therapist: You didn't feel hungry, and you used this feeling as the basis on which to decide not to have your snack.
Client: Yes that's right.
Therapist: Well this raises an interesting point. You're right, usually, hunger is a pretty good indicator of whether we need to eat or not: if we're hungry it's normally because it's been a while since we've eaten, and if we're not it's probably because we had enough at our last meal to keep us going. However, your situation at the moment is a bit different. Because you have an eating disorder, the system that governs your hunger has become dysregulated. So just for the moment, you can't rely on hunger to tell you when to eat. If you had an illness that required you to take medicine every three hours, would you take it, even if you didn't feel like it or didn't like the taste of it?
Client: Yes, I guess so, that's just what you do with medicine, isn't it?
Therapist: Ok, so eating is a bit like that, it's like your medicine. You might not feel like eating, you might not even like what you need to eat, but this doesn't mean that the best decision is not to eat because you need to eat to get better. Does that make sense?

Clients with eating disorder often have difficulty keeping the "bigger picture" in mind, tending instead to get "bogged down" by detail. The "airline pilot" metaphor (Waller's team) is used to help clients to keep focused on the bigger picture of maintaining a regular diet, even though they are worried that they have already eaten too much on a particular day, or that their weight may have changed slightly. If a client responds to having eaten "too much" on one occasion or to getting on the scales and seeing her weight has gone up, with a sudden switch to extreme food restriction, the next metaphor can be handy; it may also be helpful in relation to recovery from other long-term mental health problems.

Therapist: The problem is that you are responding to the immediate concerns, but the response is making things worse in the longer term. It is as if you were an airline pilot, flying from London to New York. You have to travel a long way, to land upon a very small piece of concrete at the other end. There are bound to be air pockets and thermals that lead the flight to have comparatively small bumps as it goes along. However, if you respond to the plane dropping a couple of feet in an air pocket by pulling back hard on the controls, the plane will jerk up sharply, and you have to push the controls forwards sharply to compensate for that. Pretty soon, the flight is made up of the plane going up and down as if it were a roller coaster. Everyone feels ill and disorientated, and it gets much harder to aim for the original target. The pilot has to learn to keep the controls straight and to react much more carefully. That ability to respond slowly and thoughtfully is one that you will need to develop if you want to reach your goal and to feel safe as you do so.

Clients with eating disorders sometimes have quite a "black and white" thinking style (see also Chapter 6, p. 113). The slow, laborious process of recovery from anorexia, with all its inherent ups and downs, can be very difficult to tolerate, and many clients tell us that if they are going to move away from their illness, they want to get it over with straight away, NOW! The problems with this are that it is not physically possible because it takes time to put on weight, and even if it were, an immediate weight gain would leave them feeling out of control, vulnerable, and likely to turn back to their anorexia for safety. The "acclimatization on the mountain" metaphor (Waller's team) can help with this:

> You are clearly very worried about the journey ahead of you if you decide to get away from being anorexic. However, we have to be realistic about the journey, and about how important it is that you do not feel that you have to do it all at once, because you will just feel out of control and probably be very tempted to give up. We need to think about this as if you were a mountaineer. Mountaineers do not aim to get to the peak of the mountain straight away. They focus on getting part way, and then taking a break

and camping on a flat piece of land. Then, when they are confident that they can take the next step, they move on. You need a chance to acclimatize on the mountain like that, so that you can move on when you are ready to take the next step. Therefore, we have to think about the journey that you have as a series of shorter steps, not as a single run.

Similarly, the "drops in a reservoir" (Treasure & Schmidt, 2007) metaphor can encourage the recognition of the value of gradual, small steps towards change when a client is finding it difficult to see any progress she is making. Within this metaphor, the anorexia nervosa thoughts are like clouds. If they encounter a mountain of strength and determination within you, they will rise and produce rain. Each act you do on behalf of your non-anorexic part, rather than your anorexic part, produces a drop of water. Over time, these drops will fill your water reservoir, giving life to your shriveled non-anorexic part. The individual battle for each drop might not be too hard to win. For example, each time you resist the urge to scrutinize calories on a label, or are victorious in adding in an extra item of nutrition, you are adding drops into your reservoir.

Perfectionism

Several important cognitive constructs in the treatment of eating disorders have been identified within the influential transdiagnostic model of Fairburn et al. (2003). These constructs are the overevaluation of eating, weight, and shape and their control, mood intolerance, low self-esteem, perfectionism, and interpersonal problems. We have already seen how metaphor can be of value in addressing issues of food and eating. The reader is referred to Chapter 6 for a discussion of metaphor use in the context of low self-esteem and mood problems, and to Chapter 11 for a more detailed look at interpersonal problems. Perfectionism, however, is a common curse afflicting those with an eating disorder, although it is also seen in many other contexts.

The continuum metaphor and the concept of "gray-scale thinking" was discussed in Chapter 6 in the context of tackling all-or-nothing thinking. Perfectionism is characterized by such black-and-white thinking processes, with self-imposed and unrelenting performance criteria such as "Any mistake means I am a complete failure." There is often an abject fear of falling short of such unattainable high standards, leading in some cases to complete paralysis. Various metaphors attempt to normalize the process of making mistakes, as in the "learning to cycle" metaphor (see Chapter 6, p. 114). It can be suggested that there is nothing wrong with actively pursuing a goal (so long as that goal is healthy and in keeping with one's other values). Rather, it is the catastrophic interpretation of falling short of these goals first time, where the problems often lie. Another metaphor that may be of use in normalizing the process of mistake-making is that of "debugging computer software." It is a known fact that, almost without exception, computer software of any significant merit cannot be written "perfectly" so it functions correctly first time. Programmers necessarily have to produce an initial version, then try running it, see where it crashes or produces errors, debug the code, test it again, and refine it through numerous such iterations, gradually approaching the standard they wish to achieve. A variant upon this is the observation that the process of producing great art, or music, frequently involves doing one or more "rough drafts" first (e.g. a pencil sketch of a scene or a scribbled notation of a melody on a stave). Indeed, most artists or musicians who tried to jump this step and write the "perfect score" or the "perfect painting" first time would surely fail to produce much of any value.

Restriction and the "rebound effect"

Another metaphor, "holding your breath," is useful with people who follow a bulimic pattern of extreme food restriction followed by binging behaviour (there are also variants that involve the function of springs or rubber bands in a similar way). It is particularly useful for helping clients to see that their inability to completely restrict their food intake for an extended period is not a personal failing but a function of their biology, and for illustrating that restriction actually sets them up for bingeing. The metaphor works well as a dialogue, as below:

Therapist: Have you ever tried to hold your breath?

Client: Yes, of course.

Therapist: How long can you do it for? A minute? Maybe a bit less or a bit more?

Client: I don't know, not that long, because you have to breathe eventually.

Therapist: That's right, in fact, it's impossible to kill yourself by holding your breath. However much you might decide that you aren't going to breathe, eventually your body takes over and makes you. What's interesting is that this is the same with food. In the same way that you have an overwhelming physical drive to breathe, you have an incredibly strong drive to eat. You can restrict your eating for a while, but eventually you're going to get so hungry that your body takes over.

Client: Ok, that makes sense.

Therapist: Let's think about when you eventually breathe after holding your breath for ages. In fact let's try it now. (Hold breath for 15 seconds or so together, and then breathe.) What did you notice about the breath you just took after holding it in for a while? Was it a normal sized breath?

Client: No, it was a big breath, sort of a gasp really.

Therapist: Right, so this is a bit like what happens when you've been restricting your food for ages and then you get so hungry that you have to eat. You don't eat just a little, or even a normal amount. Your restriction has set you up to try to eat as much food as possible, to compensate for the deprivation while you were restricting, like having to take a big gulp of air after holding your breath. So in this way, restricting your eating is actually keeping the binging going.

Eating disorders as external entities

Clients with eating disorders often find it very difficult to "see" their illness; the cognitive set—the beliefs, rules, and distortions—that come with the disorder may be perceived by a client to be her "true self," an integral and valued part of her being. Because of this, interventions that facilitate the client gaining a different, more externalized perspective on the disorder can be extremely powerful.

The "itchy jumper" metaphor (Waller et al., 2007) is a useful way to help a client to begin to see her eating disorder as separate from herself, as something that she is essentially "wearing." This metaphor goes further however, as it also provides a way of considering the pros and cons of change in the context of the "jumper" with eating disorder:

Therapist: Your eating disorder is like a jumper. When you first put it on, it keeps you nice and warm. However, it is not a "top of the range" jumper, and so after a while starts to get a bit itchy and irritating. Sometimes you might feel like taking it off, but you know that if you do you will be cold, so you put up with the itchiness. With time, however, the itchiness gets harder and harder to tolerate. It gets more and more uncomfortable, and although the jumper still keeps you warm you start to think whether there might be better ways of keeping yourself warm.

If you decide the time has come to take off your jumper it is important first to explore the other ways that you might be able to keep yourself warm. However, if you are going to go down that line, at some point you will have to take the itchy jumper off and be cold for a period while you try out some other ways of keeping warm. This might feel more uncomfortable in the short term, but in the longer term it will allow you to keep warm in an itch-free way.

If you don't feel able to change your eating behaviours at present, this might be because your jumper has not yet become itchy enough for you to want to risk being cold. If this is the case, you might need to continue wearing your jumper for a bit longer. At the same time, however, it could be helpful to explore other ways that can keep you warm, maybe ones that you can practice whilst still wearing your itchy jumper.

Other ways that an eating disorder can be metaphorically externalized are by a client developing their own visual image of their disorder. Suggesting a client try to picture her eating disorder and describe it—is it soft or hard, spiky or round, what does it sound like, does it have a face, a smell, a colour?—can be particularly powerful. Naming their eating disorder or identifying it as a particular thing or animal is a part of this, for example a client may have an

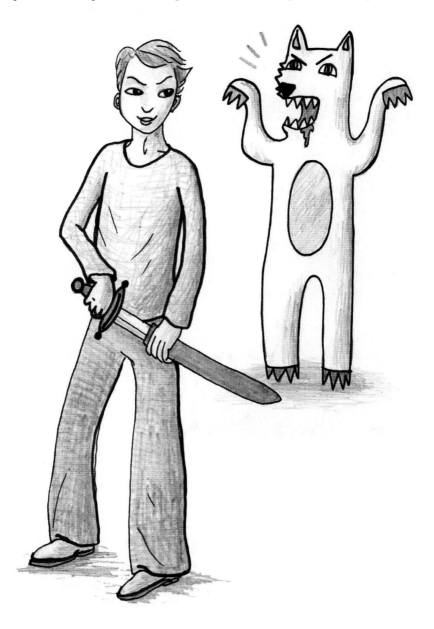

anorexic minx, or a *bulimic boa constrictor*, or the eating disorder may be seen as a *parasite*, a *monster*, an *evil elf*, or (for one client) *Tinkerbell* from Peter Pan. The idea here is that if a client can "see" her eating disorder rather than simply "being" it, it gives her more of a chance to get to know it in a different way and to start to fight against it.

Along these lines, often a very effective intervention is for a client to write letters to her eating disorder, once she has visualized and named it, as a "friend" and then as an "enemy" (Schmidt, Bone, Hems, Lessem, & Treasure, 2002). This allows the client to take the externalization a step further and to begin to engage with her eating disorder on a different basis, in a dialogue.

Narrow self-evaluation

The tendency for all-or-nothing thinking was discussed earlier. Indeed, clients with eating disorders have often become almost exclusively focused on their eating, shape, and weight as the source of their self-evaluation: it is on these criteria that they judge themselves to succeed or fail, win or lose, be good or bad. In addition to being a narrow domain, the client's extreme and inflexible goals and rules around her eating, shape, and weight mean that she is likely to experience frequent failures or live in constant fear of failure within this domain. The expansion of the range of life domains upon which a client evaluates herself is thus an important part of recovery from an eating disorder. The "all your eggs in one basket" metaphor captures both the narrowness and precariousness of this approach in a way that may lead to a productive discussion about alternatives:

Therapist: Basing the whole of your self-evaluation on your weight and how well you control your eating is a bit like putting all your eggs in one basket. If you don't reach your weight goals or follow the rules you've set yourself, this is like dropping the basket and all your eggs breaking. As well as all your eggs being in this one basket, what makes it even more difficult is that it is a very fragile basket. It is easily dropped, as the rules and goals you've set are so rigid and harsh. An alternative would be to distribute your eggs between a number of baskets. What might these be (friends, career, other interests)? What are the advantages of spreading your eggs around? What would you make the baskets out of (more flexible rules)? How could you begin to do this?

Balancing psychological and medical needs

There can be a high level of medical risk associated with an eating disorder. When a high-risk situation is identified, it may be necessary to focus care on preventing severe physical deterioration or death, and the more psychological aspects of treatment may need to be suspended until physical safety is restored. Sometimes in this situation, a client finds it difficult to see the need, for example, to suspend valued outpatient psychological therapy and be admitted to an inpatient ward, or to change from self-esteem work that the client feels is essential to her recovery, to a focus on reducing vomiting to a less dangerous level, which may be perceived as less fundamentally important.

In this kind of situation, one of our colleagues, Miriam Grover, has suggested that thinking of the eating disorder as an "uninvited guest at a party" may be valuable. If the uninvited guest comes in and sits quietly in a corner, pretty much minding her own business, a first approach might be to sit down next to her and enquire how she got in, why she's there, who she knows at the party and generally try to get an understanding of what is going on. However, if such a guest barges in and proceeds to trash the place and cause destruction, the priority will be to get her out as soon as possible and ask questions later. (Fiddling while Rome burns would not be recommended.) Nevertheless, there is an important and validating message in this metaphor. If the uninvited guest were destructive, then although you would need to get her out of your house first, you *would* still want to ask questions to understand her fully in due course— just not straight away. This can be meaningful to clients who feel they are "just a weight" to health professionals, who they may perceive as not being interested in the psychological aspects of their difficulties and overly focused on weight.

Metaphors of addiction

Eating disorders can, in some ways, be usefully seen as addictive behaviours, and this metaphor may be of use to clinicians and clients alike. Indeed, it is not uncommon for clients to speak of having an eating binge, for example, as "getting a fix." The experience of binge eating can be subjectively compulsive, "like a drug," often accompanied by a feeling of loss of control. For those with bulimia, it is also often the case that the initial episodes of vomiting were a form of experimentation, which then, over time, took on an irresistible life of their own—again not unlike many histories of drug use.

In terms of formulation, there are often other parallels. At an emotional level, the function of eating disorder behaviour may be to suppress or avoid emotion (see also the concept of mood intolerance in the approach of Fairburn et al., 2003). In substance misuse, drug, and/or alcohol use may often usefully be regarded as a reinforced behaviour that successfully suppresses or avoids aversive emotional states. Furthermore, there are parallels in terms of "denial" cognitions that permeate both eating disorders and the addictions. For example, in bulimia, there is often a belief that one can "have one's cake and eat it" (quite literally, sometimes), i.e. be able to eat anything one wants and not have to pay for it (i.e. put on weight). This is analogous to the alcoholic who minimizes his/her usage and believes that they have a strong liver, which protects them so the usual rules don't apply. Similarly, "permission-giving cognitions" may permeate the thoughts of both individuals with eating disorders and those with addictions. Examples of such permission-giving thoughts might be *"I deserve an ice-cream because I have been so good recently"* and *"It's been a hard day so I do need just one more drink."* Careful and sensitive exploration of these analogies may be useful to help free up thinking processes and take a more healthy perspective on one's motivations and thought processes, and the true impact of one's behaviours on one's wider goals. Clients may realize that they do not wish to be "chained" into their eating disorder, just as another person may long to be free of their addiction.

Summary

This chapter has explored the use of metaphor in working with clients with eating disorders. Eating disorders can "imprison" clients, "narrowing and shrinking" their lives and radically distorting the meaning and significance of food, weight, and shape. Metaphor may offer a powerful tool in exploring and helping transform these constructs. It has also been seen how metaphor may enable novel ways to address issues of perfectionism and motivation, as well as the counterproductive effects of restriction. It may offer ways to externalize and create distance from the eating disorder itself, and to help with the broadening of life perspectives that may be beneficial to the client who feels "trapped" in their disorder. Many of the metaphors in this chapter can be transplanted into other areas of clinical work, and the reader is encouraged to take them and use them as seeds of creativity in their work with clients in a variety of settings.

Chapter 11

Interpersonal difficulties

Introduction

Interpersonal difficulties are pervasive among clients whatever their specific disorder and are often an integral part of their problems, even if they are not the immediate presenting issue. Within a cognitive approach, they form three key aspects of the formulation: the early life experiences that set the stage for later beliefs and thinking styles; the current interactions with others that are interpreted and responded to dynamically in a way that may maintain or exacerbate their problems; and the interaction with the therapist, which often diverges from the collaborative stance required of CBT. While metaphors are clearly helpful to elucidate abstract processes of thinking within CBT, they also provide tools to consider the subtleties of relationships. They may provide ways to see commonalities in painful interpersonal experiences that allow clients to realize they are not alone in their suffering, and templates for imagining new relationships that may be difficult, or impossible, for clients to conjure up from their own lives.

This chapter shares a range of metaphors relevant to interpersonal difficulties that may be useful in CBT.

Parental expectations of children

Clients' early experiences of life and relationships with their parents are often identified by both clients and therapists as being crucial to their well-being. Clients frequently experience a mixture of distressing emotions relating to their relationships with their parents, including feelings of hurt and anger and sometimes guilt and shame at these feelings. This very often creates a context whereby the "cause" of a client's difficulties are either located in their parents, or in themselves, and the oscillating emotions often seem to reflect these switching attributions. Arguably, the most useful metaphors have the ability to transcend this "blame-them-or-me" conflict and help the client to understand how the origin of their problems may be more complex.

The tool kit

When working with the distressing feelings concerning relationships, special efforts may need to be made to avoid a "blame culture" within the therapy. Within CBT, the therapist may try to explain this logically in the following way: "As part of thinking about your difficulties, we need to think about the relationships and factors in your family that may be important. If we are going to understand how your problems have developed and what is keeping them going, then we need to spend some time thinking about where you live and who you live with. I want to be really clear that I am *not* saying that this is anybody's fault. We are not trying to find anyone to blame, but the important relationships in your life are important for us to think about."

A metaphor may help to clarify what is a sensitive subject to entertain. This particular example has been provided by Waller et al. (2007): "One way of

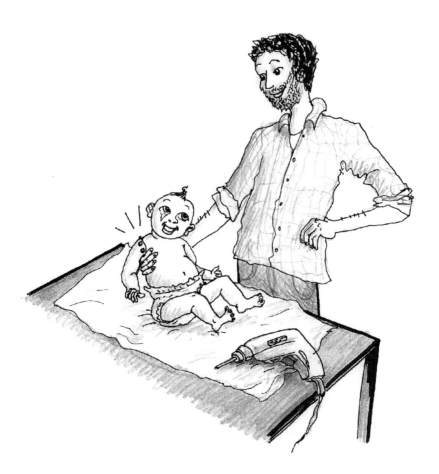

thinking about this could be in relation to a *tool box*. Each of us has a tool box, containing different tools to help us cope with everyday life. We inherit some of the tools from our parents, and we collect some along the way through our experiences of life. So, when our parents became parents, they each had different tools in their boxes. As babies and children grow up, they need differ-ent tools from their parents to help them along the way. Sometimes there are no difficulties with this—say the baby needs a spanner to fix it, and the parents have one that fits—but at other times they may not have one or have the wrong size. It is not that they don't *want* to help, but their tools are not quite right. This is because they have either not inherited the necessary tools from their own parents, or because life has not allowed them to collect the necessary tools."

The therapist would be expected to ask their client what they think of this idea before moving on further. Clearly the client's own perspective on their parents will determine whether they think that it is feasible that their parents did want to help them, yet were not able to do so in certain ways. It can open up a discussion about the differences between the intentions behind their parents' behaviour (using a tool) and the skills and knowledge available (range of tools). When applied to certain difficult interpersonal memories at the appropriate stage in therapy, this distinction may allow a helpful shift in perspective.

Guess Who's Coming to Dinner

A recurring interpersonal issue relates to independence versus dependence (Baumeister & Leary, 1995). The film, *Guess Who's Coming to Dinner*, starring Sidney Poitier, plays out this issue within a specific context: feeling indebted to one's parents to the extent that one must go along with their wishes at the expense of one's own. Poitier plays a highly educated black man, John Prentice, who, through the sacrifice of his parents, is studying to become a lawyer. He meets and falls in love with a white woman and they decide to get married. His parents demand that he calls off the engagement immediately. The turning point of the film concerns a discussion between Prentice and his father. Prentice's father points out that despite the love the couple may have for one another, the situation creates problems: Prentice will be castigated by both black and white communities, jeopardizing his future prospects as a lawyer and in doing so wasting all the hard work and sacrifice on the part of his parents. The father exclaims: "You owe it to us not to marry her and see your career through!" Prentice says: "I owe you nothing! Your sacrifice was that of free choice. I never asked you to do it!"

The client may have seen this movie already, or it could be recommended to the client if parental expectations are a recurring issue and if its content resonates for the client. It would make sense to see the whole film to provide this scene in context. Within therapy, reflection on this interaction may promote a potentially useful discussion about parental and personal choices and the rights and responsibilities that go along with these. In essence, it clarifies that the lines of responsibility can often be blurred within problematic relationships. Individuals can only be responsible for their own behaviour; conflict is created by claiming that another person holds responsibility for a decision that they were not involved in. The manner in which Poitier's character makes his case distils the logic and the moral strength of this claim, and it is one that provides a potential model for clients in this position if and when they are ready to do so.

Parents' attachment to children

In a reversal of the above situation, clients who are parents can have difficulties in separating themselves from their children, and accepting that they are autonomous beings with their own strengths and vulnerabilities. The following excerpt from 'The Prophet' by Khalil Gibran may be useful when parents feel frustrated by their children's differences from them or opposition to them and to encourage their acceptance of the limited influence they have over their children's lives.

> And a woman who held a babe against her bosom said, "Speak to us of Children."
> And he said:
> *Your children are not your children.*
> They are the sons and daughters of Life's longing for itself.
> They come through you but not from you,
> And though they are with you, yet they belong not to you.
> You may give them your love but not your thoughts.
> For they have their own thoughts.
> You may house their bodies but not their souls,
> For their souls dwell in the house of tomorrow, which you cannot visit, not even in your dreams.
> You may strive to be like them, but seek not to make them like you.
> For life goes not backward nor tarries with yesterday.
> You are the bows from which your children as living arrows are sent forth.
> The archer sees the mark upon the path of the infinite, and He bends you with His might that His arrows may go swift and far.
> Let your bending in the archer's hand be for gladness;
> For even as He loves the arrow that flies, so He loves also the bow that is stable.
>
> Gibran (1992)

In our experience, a good degree of clinical judgement is required when using literature, such as the above poem, with clients. Like any metaphor, they need to be chosen to focus on a key concern of the client that the formulation indicates relates directly to their problems. The format—a poem—will be more suitable for some clients. Then, even once provided, they are only a starting point for reflection, and it is the discussion about the meaning of the metaphor for the client that is important. In this poem, it is most likely the positive future-directed imagery that provides the power—"their souls dwell in the house of tomorrow"; "living arrows sent forth." These images may provide a constructive perspective on allowing a child's autonomy that provide alternatives to the client's existing images of their child's vulnerability and dependence. Through discussion, the therapist may help the client make the step to considering how these strong and compassionate images can then apply to the reality of their own child (see also Chapter 12).

Abuse

The sensitive and private topic of abuse lends itself naturally to metaphor. Indeed, much of the imagery within children's literature seems to allude to this unspoken experience, and help prepare children for how to cope. A brief list reveals the trauma behind many apparently palatable fairytales: the imprisonment of Rapunzel, the neglect of Cinderella, the emotional abuse of Quasi Modo, and the sadistic menace of children by the Child Catcher in *Chitty Chitty Bang Bang*. We have focused here on one particular excerpt because of the way in which it empowers the viewer to challenge their abuser. Often, adults who were abused as children still hold the conceptual framework of their abuser as a powerful person with the capacity to continue to terrorize and traumatize them, either in real life or in memory. The metaphorical scene from the *Wizard of Oz* provides a way for the client to shift perspective from the imagined "all-powerful" Wizard to the, in reality, powerless individual. In doing so, it offers an alternative mindset and can disarm the abuser by recategorizing him as an impotent impostor. In the scene, Dorothy and her friends reach the palace of the Wizard, in the Emerald City. The Wizard appears as a terrifying presence with a huge face and a booming voice. Dorothy and her friends cower in the corner, petrified with fear. At this point, someone pulls a curtain away and the Wizard is revealed as a little man working some illusionist machinery. They realize suddenly that they are not scared of him because he cannot do them any harm; he does not possess any magic, he is just a little man with a box of tricks. This vivid metaphor can provide an entry point to discuss whether the client's abuser may have similar "tricks" that gave the impression of power—tone of voice, size, vacuous threats. A "deconstruction" of the abuser in this way may facilitate the client's confidence in future interactions in real life, within role-play or through imagery rescripting.

Personal vulnerability

Some of our clients continue to feel vulnerable to attack or abuse in most of their adult lives. In our experience, clients often describe metaphors that convey this powerful felt sense. It appears fruitful to return to their metaphor throughout the therapy to try to establish how their experience of vulnerability is changing over time, and to consider ways to help reduce it. For example, one client described his most vulnerable periods as being "like a *snail without a shell*, with birds circling overhead." It was accompanied by sheer terror and a fatalistic belief that "this was it"; this was the time he would be attacked and left for dead. At other times, he talked about "crawling into his shell." This represented the times when he would engage in safety behaviours such as literally hiding, or more often, numbing himself from his own feelings of fear so that even if he was attacked, he would feel nothing. Sometimes he would use drugs, alcohol, or excessive amounts of caffeinated drinks to try to bring on this numbed state of mind, whereas other times he was frustrated by his incapacity to do so; again he returned to the snail-with-no-shell, open to attacks on its tender pink flesh.

During therapy, the client and therapist returned to this metaphor. When asked how he knew that the birds are circling over head, he said that he knew it from how vulnerable he felt without his shell. He dare not actually look to see if they were overhead for fear they would see him. This metaphor provided an entry point to behavioural experiments targeted at testing out the environment; attending to other people for a few seconds to see if they did look like they would attack him. The idea of the shell was also elaborated. If he was a snail he needed a shell; it was normal to be protected. Therefore his task was to develop a shell that he could always have with him, and that allowed him to go about his life, attending to his environment, knowing he had safety when he needed it. Some of the strategies he learned during therapy formed part of this shell: noticing his fearful thoughts and challenging them; treating himself in a caring, compassionate way, and allowing himself to take his life a step at a time without feeling highly critical towards himself. We hope this example illustrates the opportunities generated by client-centred metaphors not only within sessions, but across the course of therapy.

Conflict and criticism

The "judo" metaphor is from David Burns' bestselling book *Feeling Good: The New Mood Therapy* (Burns, 1980). Judo is a martial art that exploits the opponent's own attacks against you. For example, if your opponent tries to punch you, the skill is to use the energy behind that punch to send the attacker off balance by continuing to pull in the direction of the punch. The principle is that attacks aimed at you can be used to your own advantage. The metaphor is a great example of how to deal with criticism by actually eliciting criticism from the accuser in the same way as judo and breakaway training by actually using the momentum of your challenger's blows against themselves. The therapist can explain to the client what techniques can be used. One of these is to ask the criticizer to be more specific. This has several effects. First, it strips the criticism of its judgemental, evaluative, and overgeneralized features; "you are an idiot" becomes "you made a mistake at the decorating." Second, it catches your criticizer off guard: you are neither accepting nor denying their criticism. Third, it means that you are not escalating the situation with your own attacks: within the metaphor it replaces escalating punching and brawling with a swift

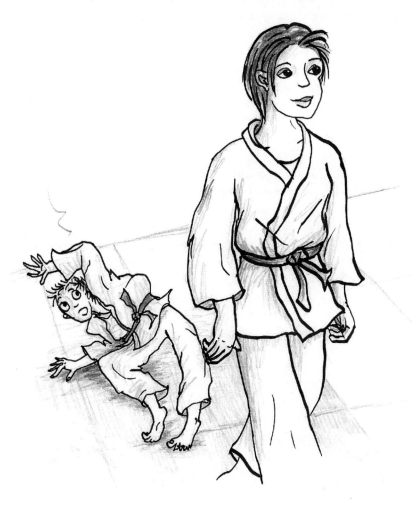

efficient use of a judo move. The judo expert can endure attacks but he does not provoke further attacks on himself. In this way, the client does not have to accept extreme criticism that is unfounded, but can show the strength to accept comments that may be a true reflection of events and may have led to frustration or disappointment. The client may even turn helpful criticism to his or her own advantage and see it as a tip of something else he or she can try out.

Scapegoating and stigma

Very often, our clients' experiences of criticism from those close to them are not isolated events. Within their family, they may have been targeted especially for sustained criticism and forced to accept a subordinated identity. A negative self-concept can often develop within the subtle ways that families interact and represent one another in their own minds. Often part of therapy involves witnessing this history, understanding how it has influenced the client's deeply held beliefs and validating the client's responses at the time. Metaphors may help to crystallize this process and show how it is part of a shared human tendency.

There are clear analogies of these toxic social processes in everyday examples. Did you ever play "It" or "The Lurgy" at school? In this child's game, if you get touched by a person who has the "lurgy" you have to run around and catch someone else who then has to do the same. This can work as an analogy for how families (or other groups) try to externally attribute blame among themselves, with each person trying to blame someone else. By seeing this process as a game, clients may be able to step back and see how childish it is. Instead of seeing their family members as powerful, critical figures, they may begin to see the circularity and pointlessness of the process. This can be extended by asking whether if this was a real illness they would do the same thing? Clearly not. This could imply that to some degree the individuals involved in the "lurgy" were not fully aware of the damaging implications of their behaviour for the client in the long term. As we see with many metaphors, it is their perspective-shifting capacities that make them particularly powerful. Nevertheless, this needs to be set in a clinical context; clients may not shift perspective when we expect them to; they may arrive at a different perspective shift to that which we had planned; they may come back the following week with their insights despite efforts by the therapist during the session. For some clients, a similar analogy may be more helpful—the "hot potato". In this example, people keep throwing a hot potato around and no one is brave or wise enough to keep hold of it, or put it aside and wait for it to cool down. In the same way, criticism and conflict tends to build up in impulsive exchanges because no individual attempts to pause to consider or clarify the criticism directed at them, or to step outside the situation for a short while. Again, this example illustrates that blame and criticism are processes that are simple and childish in nature and can be addressed and de-escalated with some simple strategies.

Social support: the spider's web

Many people with a history of mental health problems have not expanded their lives and may have avoided a variety of social experiences. They may have been brought up by their family, been to school, and had school friends and childhood interests and hobbies. However, they may have not expanded the range of people they know, or their activities and interests. Eventually elements of the family die out or move away; friends grow up, get married, and move away and the person ends up with very few people around them. Childhood activities become less relevant or no longer accessible and increasingly limited.

The next metaphor, provided by Aidan Bucknall, uses the structure of a spider's web to represent a social network. If you look at how the spider builds its web there tend to be some major cross strands that provide structural support. There are also interconnections and some lighter strands that make up the rest of the web. The structure provides two important functions. The first is as a good mesh for catching prey. The second is that, as it is well meshed, it can be damaged without completely collapsing, allowing the spider to repair parts of the web and not having to start all over again with a new web. The idea is that the spider recognizes that if it invests too much in any one strand then (a) the web won't work for catching prey and (b) it would take very little damage to destroy the web. The spider solves this by making sure that the strands are interlocked and form many connections with other strands protecting the integrity of the web. So in an individual who is isolated, with narrow social contacts and few activities or interests, a good method is to draw out the person's web. The client is asked, for example, who the important people in their lives are and about the things that they feel are important. These are plotted in a diagram shaped as a web. The client would then be asked whether their diagram is a viable web; is it one that a spider would weave? Would the web capture food? What would happen if one of the strands snapped?

Commonly, the client's web would collapse if a few strands were damaged. In this respect, the therapist can visually highlight the client's anxiety. In practice, clients such as this often show overattachment to particular people and are anxious about these attachments. This makes sense because these attachments are the strands that hold the client's web together. In order to relive

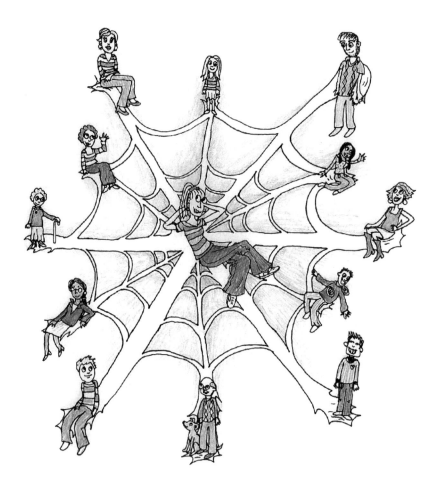

some of the anxiety, the client is asked whether they need to widen their range of activity and social relations to increase the connections and build more strands so that their web is less vulnerable. The metaphor can help clients recognize that if they have pared their lives down to the bare basics, they become very vulnerable and can easily come to "live on their nerves." It then provides them with a framework to consider the reasons for building their web up again for the sake of their own strength and resilience.

Anger, passivity, and assertiveness

Anger generally emerges from perceived unfairness or violation of one's rights within a social system. It is one of the most metaphorically rich emotions, and one most studied psycholinguistically (Kövecses, 2000). Indeed, it is virtually impossible to describe the human experience of anger without recourse to metaphor. Clients will therefore often spontaneously describe how they are "boiling" with rage, or feel like they are going to burst. Sometimes they will also say they are "inwardly" boiling, but try to "keep a lid on it." These derive from the well-studied conceptual metaphor of "anger as a hot fluid in a container" (Lakoff & Kövecses, 1987). Other common sources domains for anger include storms ("I'm a stormy person"), fire ("I'm smouldering with fury"), and forceful agents ("I'm struggling with my anger"). Very often, such metaphors are meaningful to clients not only at a verbal or imaginative level, but they will actually "feel" them bodily (e.g. "I can *feel* my temperature rising"; "My blood is going to boil"). Working therapeutically with such metaphors therefore involves a careful understanding of the meanings and embodied experiences underlying their words (see also Chapter 3, p. 46 for an example of a helpful metaphorical transformation with an angry client who believed they were a "bomb waiting to go off").

Passivity often stems from the inability of an individual to effectively stand up assertively for their rights or needs. During therapy, clients learn how to make their needs heard, and then outside the session, develop their personal goals in a way that establishes them. Prior to this, their blocked goals tend to manifest themselves as anxiety (e.g. fear of failure), depression (hopelessness concerning the pursuit of goals), or bursts of aggression (impulsive attempts to re-establish control). Often, our clients' passivity comes from trying to follow other people's rules and goals rather than their own. During therapy, clients realize that they "need to stay in their own lane" to work through their own problems rather than taking excessive responsibility for others. Some clients have particular difficulties with assertiveness, switching from passivity to anger or aggression and back again. The source of the passive behaviour is often thoughts such as "I deserve this," "It's wrong to ask for help," or "I should be able to do this." The reactive, aggressive behaviour often comes from a sense that "people are taking the piss" or a build up of resentment about being put upon. Another common problem is of people seeing themselves as very "giving" without being aware that the things they are giving may not be what the other person wants.

There are two metaphors we have encountered that seem to describe this process well and provide some new perspectives. The analogy of a "pressure cooker" is built upon the "hot fluid in a container" metaphor described earlier. This can help to illustrate the very real process of feeling stress and anger built up inside after periods of inassertiveness. We may feel stress or anger and yet do or say nothing, and so pressure builds up within us and has nowhere to go. Eventually, the pressure builds up so much that it causes us to "explode," in a burst of aggression. In order not to allow pressure to build so much that it results in an explosion, we have to find a safe way to release it. In this way, assertive behaviour can act as a "pressure valve." All pressure cookers contain a valve of this kind to prevent them from "blowing the lid off"; it is an essential design feature. This analogy can help to both justify some level of "release" of stress while also getting the client to consider the problems of experiencing aggression or panic that is out of control because of its potential impact on the self and others. What kinds of pressure valves does the client want to create in their life? How can the client learn when to engage in them?

Another useful way of discussing this is to consider the process from an interpersonal perspective: happy relationships are like a well-balanced *seesaw*. The easiest way to keep the seesaw balanced is to just put all the weight in the middle (representing compromise). But, obviously we can't always do this if people are at opposite ends. So, for everything that gets put on one end, something else must be put on the other end of "equal weight." Problems can arise because the other person gets some say in what gets put on. It must be negotiated that what is at each end is of equal weight, although it does not have to be the same object. Clients tend to be immediately aware of the equity of such an approach, and it would tend also to reflect the collaborative stance that is taken within the therapy sessions themselves.

Guilt and shame

Guilt and shame are two other central emotions that appear across many clinical presentations, as well as being familiar to all of us at times. Guilt refers to the perception that one's behaviour has transgressed one's own internal standards, and shame refers to a sense that oneself is unacceptable or bad, often in the eyes of others. Both are typically "social emotions" in the sense that the individual tends to be evaluating themselves and their actions within an interpersonal context. The person feeling guilty often believes they have been unfair or unjust to someone else, or that their behaviour has not lived up to someone else's expectations. The person experiencing shame often believes they are fundamentally unacceptable to others (although Gilbert (1998) has made a strong argument for the existence also of "internal shame" in which the emphasis is purely on how the individual feels about themselves).

As with other emotions, metaphor plays a central role in our conceptualizations, feelings, and abilities to describe and communicate such feelings to others. Therefore, we may feel "burdened" by guilt, and even sense it bodily as "weighing heavily" on us. Metaphors of guilt and dirtiness also run deep in our culture (e.g. "This is a stain on my reputation"; "I don't want to wash his dirty linen" and so forth). However, in working with guilt, across a variety of contexts, there is often a need for the clinician to tackle some of the underlying cognitive biases that fuel the guilt (e.g. Kubany, 1998). A classic example is the notion of hindsight bias, which often creeps into people's thinking processes when an undesirable outcome has occurred. This bias refers to a negative judgement about a past decision based on a later outcome, not known at the time of the decision being taken. Individuals often berate themselves for making a decision because it "caused" a bad outcome—they think they "should not" have made that decision and thus feel guilty about it. What they knew at the time becomes muddled and conflated with what they knew later (in particular the bad outcome).

This somewhat abstract notion can sometime be understood intellectually but is often hard to assimilate emotionally. One metaphor can be of help here, which can be explored collaboratively—that of the "child and the iron." Supposing a young child has never before seen an iron. They come across one, which has accidentally been left out, and they reach up to explore it and as a result have an accident (thankfully not a hugely traumatic one because the iron was not hot!). Would you be very cross with the child? Probably not, as they could not know of any dangers—it was their first encounter. But, supposing you then explained carefully to the child that they must never ever touch an iron, because it could be hot and burn them very badly. Then, if the child encountered an iron would your reaction be different towards them? Well, possibly, yes, you might be cross because they had the knowledge of danger and chose to ignore it. So what does this tell us about the link between knowledge and responsibility? A discussion along these lines can sometimes help allow a shift of perspective sufficient to begin to see properly the unfairness of the hindsight bias.

Shame, by contrast, is frequently described in terms of "hiding" or "vanishing" metaphors: the desire to bury one's head in the sand, or to be "swallowed up" by the ground. However, it is worth considering that people do use such emotion terms in a variable way, both within as well as between cultures. To ensure accurate understanding and ability to offer effective help, it may be particularly helpful to attend to the metaphorical language at play. For example, one client, when asked what her shame was like, said "I feel like I'm a speck of dirt which no one can quite get rid of." Further exploration revealed the idiosyncratic, encapsulated meanings embedded within this metaphor, which became central to the case conceptualization: of littleness, insignificance but also of nuisance, irritation, and even embarrassment to others.

Summary

In the chapter we have considered the role of metaphors in a range of interpersonal difficulties. They particularly illustrate how relationships and the relating process are represented within cognition—people have mental models for how they consider significant others in their lives. When these mental models are distilled as vivid metaphors, they may have a greater capacity for discussion and change. In the next chapter, we focus particularly on one class of relationship—between parent and child where the child rather than adult is presented to services with an ongoing difficulty.

Chapter 12

Working with parents

Introduction

This chapter focuses on the use of metaphor in working with parents of children who have psychological difficulties, particularly behavioural problems and anxiety disorders. For younger children, i.e. those under the age of about nine or ten years, there is little evidence for the effectiveness of any direct therapies, such as CBT (Cartwright-Hatton et al. 2004). On the other hand, there is now a substantial mass of evidence for the effectiveness of behavioural parent training programmes, such as *Triple P* (Sanders, 1999) and *The Incredible Years* (Webster-Stratton et al., 2004). Much of this evidence relates to the treatment of childhood behaviour problems; however, a group of clinicians and clinical researchers in Manchester, including one of us (S.C.H.), have been developing this approach for use with parents of anxious children. This chapter will describe some metaphors that the group has found useful with each of these populations.

In working with parents, and, in particular, in delivering a behavioural parent training program to groups of parents, metaphors are useful for a number of reasons. First, as is probably the case in all therapeutic modalities, the use of metaphor can illuminate a complex concept that the therapist wants to communicate to a client. However, a successful metaphor can then also provide a convenient "shorthand" for this concept, which can be re-introduced with a minimum of additional explanation, throughout the remainder of therapy. Third, when working with parents, we are sometimes dependent on the parent for transmission of concepts to their child. Providing a well-developed metaphor can give parents a simple "off the peg" means of transmitting this information, reliably and entertainingly, to their child. Finally, many clinical psychologists use metaphor when communicating difficult personal messages to parents (such as when the therapist believes that a parent's behaviour is contributing to a child's difficulties). The use of metaphor can not only help to communicate this information clearly, but can also diffuse the potentially threatening tone of the message. Examples of each of these uses are given below.

General metaphors for working with parents

Dealing with blame and responsibility

When parents come along to behavioural parent training groups, they sometimes do not arrive with a completely open mind. Some parents have been coerced into attending by professionals who have made it clear that they think the parent's skills are lacking in some regard. Others are there willingly, but have come because they suspect that their parenting skills are substandard, and that they may, in some way, be responsible for their child's difficulties. In either situation, the therapist has to work fast to build a relationship with the parent. Failure to achieve this relationship within the first session is a key cause of client dropout, which can be very high in these settings.

One issue that most therapists choose to tackle as a matter of urgency is perceptions of who is "to blame" for the child's problems. This is a tricky area to navigate because, while the therapist needs to develop a warm, accepting, noncritical relationship with the parent, they also need the parent to leave the session having decided to begin making some changes to their parenting. There seems to be a high correlation between the trickiness of the message and the number of metaphors that have evolved to communicate it, and this tricky area is no exception. Several useful metaphors are in circulation.

Dr Caroline White has developed the clever "behaviour CAKE (causal attribution and knowledge-based explanation)" metaphor for discussing issues of causality with parents. In this metaphor, a *cake recipe* (flour, butter, eggs, sugar, chocolate chips) is written up on the white board. The parents are invited to shout out the ingredient that makes the cake "taste nice." Inevitably, someone says "the chocolate chips," and this triggers a discussion of what the cake would taste like if a dull ingredient, such as the flour, were left out. The message in this metaphor is that lots of ingredients must come together to make a cake, much as lots of ingredients must come together to make a child's personality. At this point, the group brainstorms a list of "ingredients" that go into making a child; genes, school, friends, past experiences, health, etc. are elicited and written on the board, as, hopefully, is "parents." A discussion follows, focussing on which of these many ingredients are amenable to change. The conclusion (helped along by the therapist) is that many of the factors that go into making children the way that they are, are not malleable. In fact, the only thing that parents really have any control over is the parenting that they provide for their child. In this way, the therapist is making explicit that he or she does not blame the parent for the child's difficulties, but does see them as a very important person in helping their child to progress.

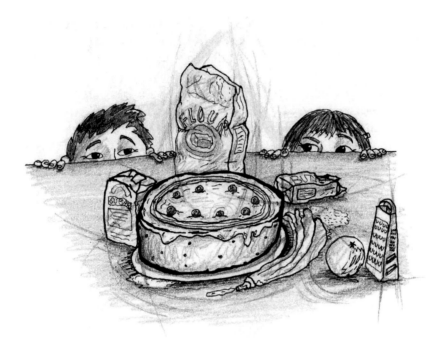

A second metaphor that is often used in context of blame and responsibility is the "car crash" metaphor (see also Chapter 4, p. 55). Most people will know someone who has been involved in a minor bump in their car. Often these accidents happen to completely blameless drivers—someone in the car behind is not paying attention, and drives into the back of your car at traffic lights. In this case, who is to blame for the accident? Clearly it is not our poor parent, but the person who drove into them. That may well be the case, but who is responsible for getting the damaged car to a garage, dealing with the insurance company, hiring a spare car until theirs is fixed? It is, of course, our blameless parent. They were not responsible for the bump, but they have to sort it out. That's life, and that's what it's like being a parent. It's not your fault that your child has these difficulties, but you are the best person in the world to fix it for your child. A variant on this theme is the "sick child" metaphor. One of us has used this with some families for whom it felt appropriate. The parent is asked to think about a child who has diabetes, or another chronic illness, such has asthma. Whose fault is the diabetes? It is no one's fault. But who has to take the child to hundreds of appointments, give the child their injections, cook special food for the child, etc. Yes, it's our poor parent again, and managing childhood behaviour problems/anxiety is no different. It is probably no individual person's fault that the child has these problems, but it's the parent who is the best person to step in and fix it. However, you would not expect the parent of a diabetic child to just know how to do the injections, and what food the child can and cannot eat. Parents of diabetic children get special training and coaching, and lots of support from professionals. We think that parents of children with psychological difficulties deserve special training and support too.

A final metaphor for dealing with the blame/responsibility issue is the widely used "washing machine" metaphor. What is more complicated? A washing machine or a child? Of course, a child is a million times more complicated. So why is it that a washing machine comes with a 200-page manual, complete with trouble-shooting section and phone helpline and a child does not? We think that this is a terrible shame, and that parents should think of our courses as the manual for their beautiful, complicated child.

The parenting pyramid

Moving on through the parenting course, and again, dangerous waters are encountered. The basis of most behavioural parenting programs is that children will respond to reinforcement programmes. If their behaviour (good or bad) results in reinforcement, they will put *more* energy into producing that behaviour in future. If their behaviour (good or bad) does not result in reinforcement they will put *less* effort into producing this behaviour in future. Therefore, parents need to shift towards giving reinforcement (particularly praise and reward) to behaviours that they do like (doing your homework, playing nicely with your sister, going to sleep on your own). At the same time, parents need to give less reinforcement to behaviour that they do not want (e.g. tantrums, excessive reassurance seeking). However, this shift in reinforcement patterns needs to be managed quite carefully. Parents need to start giving lots of attention and other reinforcement to behaviour that they do like, *before* they start trying to extinguish behaviours that they don't like. If they do not do things in this order, then the child will find that they are getting very little reinforcement for any of their behaviours, and progress will be difficult and slow. This often feels very counterintuitive to parents, who are keen to find rapid solutions to their children's difficult behaviour.

Carolyn Webster-Stratton has come up with a very useful metaphor for explaining why things are done in this order to parents. Her programmes introduce parents to the "parenting pyramid." This pyramid has several layers, each labeled with a key parenting technique that will be taught in the course. It begins with parent–child play at the bottom, and moves up, through praise and reward, towards removal of reinforcement for unwanted behaviour, through effective limit setting, and into Time Out. The pyramid metaphor is an apt one, as there is strong evidence to suggest that parents who put most of their effort into the smaller top layers—i.e. into punishing or removing positive reinforcement for children's difficult behaviours are more likely to have children with behavioural difficulties. The pyramid is used to demonstrate that the parent's biggest efforts need to be directed towards the large, stable foundations of the pyramid—i.e. towards building a relationship with the child (through play) and reinforcing desired behaviours using praise and reward. Conversely, parents should be directing less effort (and doing it later in the programme) towards the smaller layers of punishment and removal of reward at the top of the pyramid.

Dr Caroline White has pushed the "parenting pyramid" metaphor further: instead of using a diagram of the pyramid, she has produced a physical pyramid, made out of children's blocks. She invites a parent to come and try to build the pyramid upside down (i.e. with the punishment and time out layers at the bottom, and the play and praise and reward layers at the top). It is, of course, impossible, and just falls down, no matter how hard people try. She uses this physical metaphor to reinforce the message that good parenting starts with a strong foundation of relationship-building play, and the praising and rewarding of desired behaviours. The metaphor is also useful in explaining to the impatient parent why they have to wait to near the end of the course for advice on how to deal directly with difficult, unwanted behaviours in their children.

Physical metaphors

One of the present authors, working on the PACMan (Parents for Anxious Children—Manchester) trial of a cognitive-behavioural parenting-based intervention for young anxious children, has used a number of *physical* metaphors. These are metaphors where a physical movement is used to represent the concept that is being taught. We find that having cues that are visual, as well as verbal is very helpful for parents. We think that it keeps things interesting and probably targets a different type of memory, increasing the chances that concepts will be remembered over time. Examples of physical metaphors are described in the sections below.

Metaphors for parents of anxious children

Break it down

One of our key physical metaphors is used to remind parents to "Break it Down!" "Break it Down" is a technique that we teach to parents to help them to remember that children need to learn new skills (including conquering fears) little by little. We teach parents to break new skills into a series of very small steps that children learn in order. The parents reinforce each step using praise and reward, and it is very useful for increasing children's prosocial behaviour, and excellent for conquering fears and phobias. However, it is tempting for parents, frustrated by slow progress in behaviours that many of their children's peers will already have mastered, to leap ahead, and expect too much of their child. We teach parents to break each new skill down into a series of steps.

On one occasion, in an uncharacteristic moment of frivolity, Dr. Stewart Rust introduced his explanation of "Break it Down" with a hip-hop style arm maneuvre (it defies description here—ask a teenager, if you are struggling), much to the amusement of the parents and other therapist. The little "Break it Down" arm maneuvre stuck, and for the remainder of the course, whenever a parent needed to be reminded to keep steps really small, the action would be repeated. Parents even began to use it themselves, and it became a motif for the group. We now use it for all groups: it has become a shorthand for quite a complex message, but one that parents universally like and remember.

The tale of the dragon in the mountain

In running groups for parents whose children have anxiety disorders, a number of key psychological constructs need to be learned and fully understood by parents. One such construct is the idea that avoidance of feared stimuli is a powerful maintainer of anxiety. It is absolutely crucial to the success of the therapy that parents understand and believe this. Therefore, fairly early in treatment, the story of "The Dragon in the Mountain" is shared with parents. It can also be used effectively with children and adolescents themselves. The story tells of a group of villagers who live at the foot of a remote volcano in a far-off land. They live a happy life, as the slopes of the volcano are lush and fertile, and the villagers need to do no more than hop up the volcano and fill their baskets with beautiful foods and then spend the rest of the day sleeping off their feast. But then one day, a terrible event befell the villagers. There was a dreadful storm. The rain lashed the mountain side, the thunder rolled and the lightning cracked, silhouetting the volcano against the black, stormy sky. The villagers were terrified and wondered what on earth was happening. Then, one of the village elders piped up "ahhh, it is the dog in the mountain. He is angry with us for taking his food." The villagers were terrified and the next day, nobody dared go up the volcano to get food. Then next day came, and still nobody would go up the volcano, and the next week came, and the next month came, and the next year came, and still nobody would dare go up the mountain. And as the months rolled by, the rumors grew, as rumors will, and it stopped being a dog in the mountain, and became a lion in the mountain, and then soon it became a dragon in the mountain, and before long, it was a fire-breathing, baby-eating dragon in the mountain and there was *no way* anyone was going up there to get food. But then, the unthinkable happened. The rains failed, and the few meager crops that the villagers had been managing to grow in the thin soil at the bottom of the volcano, failed. The villagers were starving, and called a meeting to decide what to do.

At this point, parents are asked what the villagers should do. Someone will usually shout "go up the mountain", and the story continues. The villagers

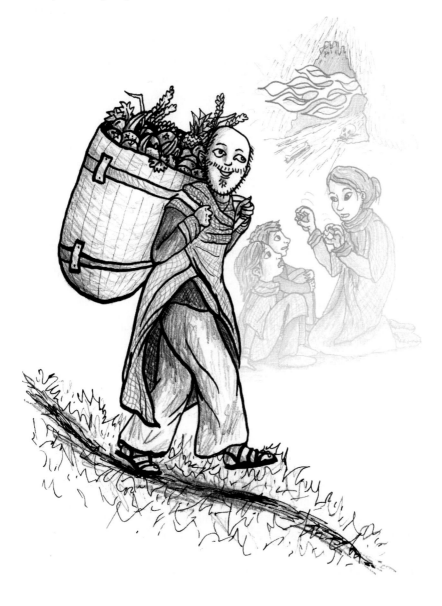

decided that they should send someone up the mountain to try to get some food, as they were doomed to starvation if they did not. So an old man set off up the volcano. His heart was beating and his chest was tight, but he kept walking, and he kept walking, and eventually he neared the top of the volcano. But just as he reached the top of the volcano, THERE WAS A GINORMOUS...... Oh how old are you lot? There are no such things as dragons. He filled his baskets with food, took it back to the villagers, who all had an enormous feast, and lived happily ever after. The moral of the tale, as the parents and children who hear it all agree, is that if you are scared of something, you have to go up the mountain; you have to test out your fears. The second moral of the tale is that if you don't do this quickly, your fears grow and grow, until they are terrifying.

Once elicited, these two morals are then revisited repeatedly during the course of the intervention. However, instead of having to repeatedly remind parents of the "deleterious role of avoidance in the aetiology and maintenance of anxiety," we can just say "anyone remember the Dragon in the Mountain?" We also use another physical metaphor to bolster our second moral from this tale. When explaining that, over time, the villagers' fears grew and grew, the therapist gradually outstretches their arms, until they are at full stretch. After telling the story, and when asking the parents to guess the moral of the tale, the therapist cues the answer by outstretching their arms as he or she did when telling the story. This always cues the correct answer from parents, and it then becomes a useful physical shorthand for the effect of avoidance on the growth of fears and phobias, which is used for the remainder of the intervention.

Parenting hotspots

Another message that can be difficult to transmit sensitively to anxious families is the role of the parents' anxiety in their children's difficulties. There is increasing evidence that many fears and phobias have no traumatic aetiology, and are, instead, learned by children hearing threatening information from others, or vicariously by watching others be scared (e.g. Field, 2006). This route is particularly likely if the child has an anxious parent who is frequently fearful. In working with anxious parents, it is important that they are aware of the impact that their anxiety can have on their child, but also important that these (often quite sensitive) parents do not feel blamed and overly responsible for their child's difficulties. On the contrary, most of these parents are in need of a boost in their parenting confidence. In order to manage this situation, we have developed a number of metaphors to help parents contextualize and be accepting of their limitations, but to be ready to make changes.

The first is the concept of the "parenting hotspot." The "parenting hotspot" is an aspect of the individual's personality that comes along and puts a "spoke in the wheel" of their parenting. Some time is spent discussing personality, and getting an agreement that we all have good and bad bits to ours. The therapist then explains that *all* parents (yes, even expert superparents off the telly) have bits of their personality that come along and stick spokes in the wheels of their parenting. This is human nature, and the best parents are not those without hotspots, but those who know where their hotspots are. The discussion turns to us each identifying our own hotspots (and if you are anxious, your anxiety is an obvious first place to look) and thinking about what we can do to

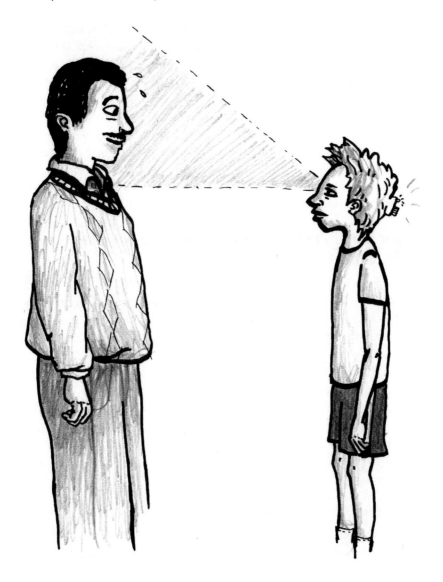

minimize their impact. This metaphor is very successful in allowing parents to acknowledge difficulties in their parenting without feeling that they are announcing that they are inadequate.

The anxious child's radar

A second issue here is that, if you have an anxious child, then you have to try harder than most parents to contain your parenting hotspots. An average, robust child can probably cope with a parent who occasionally gets visibly stressed, or catastrophizes publicly from time to time. For an anxious child, however, this is a real problem. These children can pick up fears and worries from the slightest demonstration of parental emotion, or the smallest throw-away comment, and their parents have to be extremely careful not to display their anxiety inappropriately. The therapist advises these parents, while washing their child's hair later that day, to look closely at their scalp. It is a little known fact that anxious children, just up from their crown, have an enormous *radar* that can detect threat, fear, and general stressing-out at up to a thousand paces. The therapist gravely warns parents that if they find this radar in their child's hair (and to be honest, most of them know if their child has one of these without even looking) they must try to be on best behaviour, and try extremely hard not to convey their own fears and worries to their child.

Zipper mouth, Botox face, and the Oscar-winning performance

Following on from the discussion of the anxious child's radar, it can help such parents to try to cover up their fear if they find themselves in a frightening situation with their child. We encourage parents to try three techniques: the "zipper mouth," the "Botox face," and the "Oscar-winning performance."

Zipper mouth (provenance unknown)

The "zipper mouth" is useful for parents who find themselves worrying out loud in front of their child. When they hear themselves about to say something that could convey fear information to their child, parents are simply asked to imagine that they have a zip on their mouth (like Zippy from the 1980s British TV series "Rainbow"), which they can zip up, to stop any words coming out.

Botox face

In situations where the parent's body language or facial expression gives away information that he or she might be detecting threat in the environment, we ask parents to use "Botox face," which is a metaphor coined by Dr Stewart Rust. For "Botox face," parents are encouraged to emulate a famous Hollywood actress who (for legal reasons, we do not wish to name her here) has had so much Botox that she cannot show a single flicker of emotion. Parents are asked to imagine that they cannot move a muscle in their face, so they are not giving away clues that they are frightened.

The Oscar-winning performance

The "Oscar-winning performance" is a similar but slightly more advanced technique to Botox face, and was originally invented by Dr. Caroline White for use with parents who were struggling to ignore their children's tantrums. In its original form, it is used to help parents to cover up their emotions (anger, amusement, etc.) when they are trying to extinguish unwanted childhood behaviour by ignoring it. However, when working with anxious families, we have adopted this metaphor to encourage parents to cover up their own anxiety when they are pushing their child to do something brave. So, when the parent is feeling anxious, they are asked to produce an "Oscar-winning performance" of someone who is cool and calm, and happy. It is unclear whether parents actually manage to cover up their fear by employing this technique. However, the use of this metaphor acts as an "aide memoire" to the parent, and helps to reinforce the very important but troubling message that children can often learn to be afraid by watching their parents.

We have employed these techniques with parents coming along to PACMan groups, and with other parents who report experiencing significant levels of anxiety, and many have reported their usefulness in reducing their modelling of anxiety to their children. One parent (who was receiving help for her anxious child) had a serious fear of flying. We taught her these techniques in the run-up to their summer holiday, which would be the child's first trip on an aeroplane. This mum did a great job of "zipper mouth" in the days before the trip, confining her worrying to times when the child was out of earshot. On the day of the flight, she did an "Oscar-winning performance" of someone who was calm and happy, and on boarding the plane, as well as making sure that someone else was actually dealing with the child, she did "Botox face," covering up any grimaces, lip-biting and frowning, in an attempt to stop transmission of her distress to the child. The result was excellent—the child, who was normally very sensitive to her mother's distress, and who normally got very upset as a result, enjoyed the flight and shows no sign of having learned her mother's fear.

We have also found these techniques useful for parents who are dealing with children who display high levels of difficult behaviour. Parents are taught to ignore (withdraw all reinforcement from) their child when the child is engaging in undesirable behaviours, such as tantrums or nagging. Although parents usually internalize the concept fairly readily, they find it very difficult to put into practice. We often see parents talking to their children ("I'm ignoring you!") or laughing at their children's behaviour when they are meant to be ignoring. For parents who find this skill difficult, zipper mouth, Botox face, and the Oscar-winning performance techniques can also be very helpful.

Once again, each of these metaphors is also physical as well as verbal. The therapist will demonstrate each technique (in as dramatic and overblown way as they can muster) and when the technique is required subsequently, it is often suggested simply by means of the physical metaphor (for instance the therapist mimes zipping her mouth, or produces the "Botox face"). In doing this, the parent can be cued to remember what they should be doing without having to be told, which is always a preferable means of learning a new behaviour.

Summary

In summary, there are very many metaphors that can be used to convey complex or emotionally difficult messages to parents. Some of these have the capacity to help parents to reframe their child's problems in a more balanced and flexible way and to take the appropriate level of responsibility. Others are memorable images that help to guide them to utilize more temporary strategies, for example in circumventing the transmission of fear. Yet one of the most useful things about metaphors is that they can be fun, which is rarely a bad thing in a therapeutic setting, whether children are involved or not!

Chapter 13

Clinical art and clinical science of metaphor in CBT: future directions

Introduction

Is a bridge a work of art or a work of science? Monet, Wordsworth, and Isambard Kingdom Brunel might have rather different answers to this question, and it is doubtless the case that the frontiers of many disciplines, including art, poetry, architecture, and structural engineering have all been pushed back by the subject of the humble bridge. But the question is ultimately a silly one. Bridges are quite clearly the stuff of both art and science.

So what of cognitive bridges? In the preceding chapters we have set forth, unapologetically, our belief in the potential for metaphor to assist and enrich the delivery of CBT. We have not only presented a wide range of metaphors, but have made many suggestions as to how to use them skilfully—the "clinical art" of using metaphor perhaps. But at present we have little hard "data" on which to base our assertions. So what is the scientific context in which we feel able to make such claims? And how might we wish for this picture to evolve?

Predicting the future

Predicting the future is like playing pin the tail on the donkey. We know what we would like to happen, but cannot see where we are going. As a result, we run the risk of making hilarious mistakes, and might find ourselves ridiculed by those who aren't wearing a blindfold except that the metaphor breaks down there, because of course we are all blindfolded when it comes to predicting the future.

Nevertheless, we would like to think that it is slightly easier predicting directions than events. Like economists, we also have the possibility that our predictions might influence the turn of events. Markets can rise or fall on the basis of economic predictions, which may be flawed or not. The same is the case with psychological therapy and the use of metaphor; having provided an account of how metaphor is and might be used in cognitive therapy, we intend to finish by seeking to influence how things progress from here in terms of research and clinical practice.

The theoretical model set out in Chapter 2 needs to be developed, tested, and refined. As is usual for cognitive theories, it involves "black boxes," which can, in principle, be further broken down and the processes involved further specified, examined then tested using both descriptive and experimental methods. Clinically useful theories are like extended metaphors; they can be used to explore ideas, aid understanding, and sometimes throw up new ideas or implications, which can first be tested in the laboratory of clinical practice and then subject to the harsher scrutiny of detailed empirical investigation.

However, the clinical examples used in this book were mostly not generated by this theory, although the person generating them usually had a theory in mind. Many represent the synthesis of theory and practice of particular therapists or groups of therapists, drawing upon preexisting theoretical models of emotion in general and emotional disorders in particular and seeking to illustrate them to clients and colleagues as clearly as possible. Their development, evolution, and successful application are examples of the way in which effective cognitive therapy has developed as a skilful blend of clinical theory, clinical art, and clinical science. This combination is of course not necessarily unique to cognitive therapy, but has been refined and fully integrated into the cognitive approach in ways not seen in other types of psychotherapy. The whole process is helped by a theme running through cognitive therapy and this book; good therapy is about helping people to better understand *how their world really works*. Metaphors are examples that aid such understanding, and reflect alternative views of how the world works using real world examples. The real world of evidence-based psychotherapy is about the artful application of science in the clinical context.

Clinical art and clinical science

The truly great theoreticians responsible for the development of psychotherapy (people such as Sigmund Freud, Aaron T. Beck, Joseph Wolpe, and several more recent CBT theoreticians) all had in common that they began as clinicians who carefully listened to their clients, and in doing so identified key phenomenological factors. They used what they heard and understood to make more systematic sense of psychopathology in terms of generalizable principles; in doing so, they also took into account previous thinking, although often did so in a way which transformed it to produce a "paradigm shift." The history of the science of psychotherapy, however, makes it clear that such attempted paradigm shifts are insufficient to produce real changes in understanding and client benefit. Further fruitful direction and development has required not only that others adopt the "new" theory in their clinical practice, but also that it gain further direction from a range of research strategies, including but not confined to outcome research. Without this additional input and development, psychotherapeutic schools run the risk of becoming metaphorical or real cults that "evolve" only through pronouncements of the leadership or by a process of internecine strife.

Mostly, however, behaviour therapy and subsequently cognitive therapy/CBT have followed a different pathway, characterized in terms of the use of "empirically grounded clinical interventions" (Salkovskis, 2002). Often the starting point has been the skills of an individual "leader," but that person or group focussing their attention on the way clinical practice is informed by and informs clinical science. This type of development has not neglected the importance of clinical art; the reality is that what clinical and theoretical "leaders" in CBT are able to specify is specified by them, then expanded upon by those who follow and critically evaluate their work; sometimes this means the partial dismantling, modification, or replacement of the theoretical edifice, which formed the starting point for an approach. Both whole packages of treatments and their components are empirically scrutinized; data talks. The application of metaphor to CBT represents just such a component, and as such can be developed further through consideration of the overarching theory, and can in turn inform theoretical developments.

Empirically grounded clinical interventions

All current approaches to psychotherapy are underpinned by more or less specific theories. Over the last two decades, cognitive-behavioural approaches have not only developed general strategies for change, but also refined the specific understanding of both transdiagnostic processes and the more specific processes characteristic of particular problems. These developments have arisen from empirical research into both psychopathology and treatment. This highly flexible approach has the capacity to examine the specific mechanisms and variations required in treatment, such as the use of metaphor.

Note that these developments incorporate, but are not confined to, "evidence-based" approaches or "empirically supported treatments" as presently defined. Empirical grounding emphasizes the importance of retaining "science" element as part of the essential combination of "clinical art" and "clinical science" (see also Chapter 4, p. 72).

A major part of the importance of *empirical grounding* rather than *evidence based* or *empirically supported* approaches lies in the prospects for future development of better psychological treatments as opposed to the continued application of well-established approaches. The concept of empirical grounding encompasses elements of theory, clinical phenomenology, studies examining basic psychological science, and outcome data (Salkovskis, 2002). We consider that the use of this approach will allow refinement and progression of our understanding on how metaphor works and how it can best be incorporated into therapy. Figure 13.1 shows the main factors involved.

Many of the procedures we use clinically today are grounded not in randomized controlled trials of therapy packages, but rather in experimental studies that focus on two main issues. First, studies that identify the factors likely to be involved in the maintenance of a specific disorder, symptoms, and clinical presentations, and that could therefore usefully be modified in the course of treatment. Such experimental studies vary from very precise laboratory investigations that seek to dissect an aspect of psychopathology in ways related to the phenomenology of the problem (Clark and Teasdale, 1982) through to field experiments in which the controls are less precise but ecological validity is built in (Rachman et al., 1976; Salkovskis et al., 1999). This type of strategy has been described in considerable detail elsewhere (Clark, 1999). A further contribution is made by other research, including work on individual differences, criterion group comparisons, and epidemiological studies.

Second, it is possible to draw upon experimental studies that clarify how specific procedures or factors can be used in order to optimize treatment interventions. Such studies can involve investigations in nonclinical samples, and it seems likely that research on metaphor would benefit from experimental work of this kind. Experimental studies, fueled by clinically derived "hunches," theories of psychopathology or derived from basic psychology, can and do help introduce innovative features into practice. Translating such work into

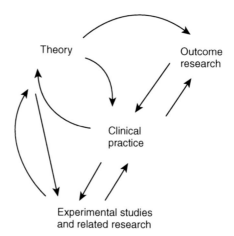

Fig. 13.1 Clinical science: empirically grounded clinical interventions.

clinical practice uses the technology of single case experimental design (Hersen & Barlow, 1976), which allows the creative application of a range of controls for threats to internal and external validity in highly flexible ways.

We must not, then, make the mistake of assuming that conducting the randomized controlled trial (RCT) (or meta-analysing a collection of them) is somehow the real science or even that it is the best type of finding (the metaphorical "gold standard"). The notion of empirical grounding allows the clinician the flexibility to go where narrowly conceived evidence based approaches cannot.

Within this approach, treatment *principles* are based on scientifically framed and evaluated theory of the maintenance of the specific problem. Treatment *procedures* are based on the best evidence about (a) the treatment package and (b) components that may be added or modified. Both *principles* and *procedures* are refined through a combination of clinical observation and theoretical and experimental development. The social and cultural context should form part of the understanding of empirically grounded clinical interventions (EGCIs). Such treatments are not only flexibly grounded in a range of evidence, but also make the gathering of evidence an intrinsic part of clinical practice.

Evaluating the use of metaphors requires such an approach, as metaphor-based cognitive therapy (MBCT) is unlikely to become a separately useful psychotherapy; as this book has illustrated, metaphors are embedded in the practice of CBT as a way of making sense of unhelpful meanings and allowing the consideration of new and more helpful meanings. It seems likely that, at least in some individuals, the use of metaphor will be a particularly effective way of making sense of what is happening and changing meaning and therefore reducing distress and psychopathology.

Fruitful avenues for research

Conceptual frameworks

As McMullen (2008) somewhat depressingly observes, much has been made of metaphor in psychotherapy but little has been learned. The literatures of basic research and applied research have evolved separately and have relatively little in common (see McCurry & Hayes, 1992 for a review). Metaphor has been extensively investigated and researched in the laboratories of cognitive science and linguistics—and much has been established, for example about the processes of metaphor comprehension, from these perspectives (e.g. Glucksberg, 2008). However, at least two factors have prevented a similarly successful development of research in the field of therapy. First, there is currently a gulf between the conceptual frameworks employed in such lab studies and the theoretical frameworks typically employed in CBT, such as Beck's notion of schemata. Clinical researchers may need to use theories that bridge both domains such as fundamental theories of cognition used to explain CBT (e.g. Teasdale & Barnard, 1993), or control theories that reflect the mechanistic and embodied nature of the construction of meaning including metaphor (e.g. Powers, 1973, 2005).

Another factor, highlighted by McMullen (2008), is that metaphor in therapy is highly contextualized. It occurs typically in the context of an interpersonal exchange between two parties, with different backgrounds, sets of experiences, and styles of learning (and even senses of humour). A decontextualized research paradigm that adopts an overly narrow focus upon the cognitive components of a given metaphor, therefore, may result in missing the essence of why that metaphor was helpful to the client on that occasion.

The theoretical model set out on page 21 seeks to capture what we believe may be the most important aspects of what is clearly both a cognitive phenomenon and a pragmatic interpersonal process, under the headlines of activation, elaboration, synthesis, and reframe. This model should be explored and if necessary refined. Ultimately a model such as this is only of use if it is capable of making valuable predictions, for example of the type of metaphors and process of application of such metaphors, which are likely to be particularly useful in therapy. Therefore, to this end, a number of different research approaches might be useful, which are outlined below.

Clinicians' use of metaphors in clinical practice

Anecdotally, it seems that metaphor is popular among many clinicians. However, it is not known the extent to which cognitive therapists actually use metaphor in therapy, or the manner in which they do so. Descriptive studies both on clinician self-report and actual recordings of therapy could be used to identify this. Several questions could usefully be asked. Is there a clear rationale for the use of a given metaphor and are the meanings consistent with the conceptualization or underpinning theory? Has the metaphor originated from the therapist or the client? What is the mode of delivery—didactic or Socratic? To what extent have the implications been followed through—e.g. for future client behaviour? Many of these issues are not straightforward to operationalize, without running the risk over being too reductionist and ignoring the context in which metaphors are employed, which is likely to be hugely important (McMullen, 2008).

Clients' experience of metaphor

Clients' experience of the use of metaphors in therapy (concurrent with therapy and/or retrospectively) could be examined in descriptive studies.

Initially, some qualitative analyses of clients' experiences of metaphor within cognitive therapy might allow us to validate, and indeed refine what we have proposed to be the key constructs and themes in the model.

The claim made in this book that metaphors assist memory could be examined (our experience being that clients sometimes recall illustrative metaphors and their meaning better than diagrammatic formulations). The use of actual or role-played therapy tapes in which metaphors are used or not, or different types of metaphor, with both understanding and memory subsequently being assessed, would extend this type of research. Factors such as vividness, imageability, and distinctiveness could be examined to determine the importance of such variables in creating effective metaphor.

While we do not consider this likely, we should be mindful of another possibility, one which is considerably less "cognitive." The rhetorical use of metaphor, in other arenas of life such as politics, can lend an impressive and convincing air of authority to a speaker. It is therefore important to know whether metaphor in therapy could be effective by virtue of the rather nonspecific effect of granting the therapist some form of elevated status. Again, this argues that research into metaphor should take into account the broader contextual factors as well as any specific cognitive hypotheses. To this end, ratings of therapist credibility, mastery, and other therapy relationship factors might usefully be examined.

It would also be valuable to explore the extent to which clients can flexibly apply a newly acquired metaphor. For example, it is all very well relating to a concept such as rumination by considering it as "spirals of spaghetti needing to be untangled"—but will this then translate into the client being able to draw upon this metaphor once "out of the therapy room," or in a slightly different set of circumstances. Will it enable the client to curtail or reduce the frequency of their rumination? Innovations may be helpful to explore here, like Otto's (2000) description of offering take-home cards with metaphorical icons on each side, a "shovel" and a "ladder" (see Chapter 4, p. 62).

Experimental studies

Experimental studies of the type described earlier could be used in a range of ways, not only to examine the impact of metaphor but also to examine the extent to which individual differences impact on the therapeutic value of metaphor, and the way different types of metaphor are received by different people. For example, the model suggests that certain cognitive tasks are necessary to process metaphor, including mental switching between domains, and being able to hold different concepts together in awareness. Therefore, it may be that people high on the autistic spectrum, older/younger people, people high and low on cognitive flexibility may benefit to different degrees depending on the properties of the metaphor and how it is introduced. Given that many of the metaphors used are transdiagnostic in their application, the impact of particular types of metaphors across different diagnostic groupings could also be examined.

There are a range of possible studies where both clinical and nonclinical participants could receive information of the same kind presented in the context of a straight fact, pictorially assisted (descriptive) and metaphor-assisted and their impact on memory, emotion, and conceptual change compared.

At a more detailed level, the extent to which the use of metaphor impacts differentially on memory at encoding versus retrieval would be informative.

The range of metaphors include those with a strongly emotional content as well as those which are more emotionally neutral; the impact of the emotional content of metaphor in different contexts would lend itself well to experimental investigation. Posttraumatic stress disorder would seem a particularly appropriate area for such research. Anecdotally, clients who have a tendency to dissociate when confronted by threatening issues seem to find processing therapy material better through emotionally salient material not directly connected with their traumatic memories, including metaphor. Within an experimental paradigm, the metaphorical nature of presented material could be varied (metaphorical versus literal) while the emotional content is kept the same, and the impact on their effective reappraisal and subsequent intrusions examined.

Summary

This chapter has set forth the context within which to consider how to progress scientifically with the study of metaphor in cognitive therapy. The notion of empirically grounded clinical interventions is an important one and helps us to think about the range of flexible research strategies at our disposal, and which have benefited many other areas of development in CBT. Also, we must also not ask overly narrow questions and neglect the contextual dimension to metaphor use. Metaphors, as described in this book, are embedded into the therapeutic dialogue. The process may be as important as the content.

We have also outlined a small selection of the types of research, which could be used to examine the use of metaphor in therapy. As with the rest of CBT, we will benefit from a greater understanding of the way in which treatment strategies such as metaphor impact on the cognitive system and how they might be helpful in allowing people to choose to change. One thing is certain; that the mutual endeavours of research and clinical practice, and the integration of clinical art and clinical science in ways described in this chapter and this book will improve our ability to understand and be understood in treatment. We believe that continued progress in these areas will, without exception, improve the quality of life for those who seek help from us.

References

Abraham, K. (1911/1953). Notes on the psycho-analytical investigation and treatment of manic-depressive insanity and allied conditions. In K. Abraham (Ed.), *Selected papers on psychoanalysis*. New York: Basic Books.

APA (1994). *Diagnostic and statistical manual of mental disorders* (4th ed.). Washington D.C.: American Psychiatric Association.

Baumeister, R.F., & Leary, M.R. (1995). The need to belong: Desire for interpersonal attachments as a fundamental human motivation. *Psychological Bulletin, 117*, 497

Beardsley, M.C. (1972). Metaphor. In P. Edwards (Ed.) *The Encyclopedia of philosophy (Vol. 5)*. New York: Macmillan.

Beck, A.T. (1967). *Depression: Clinical, experimental, and theoretical aspects*. New York: Harper & Row.

Beck, A.T. (1976) *Cognitive therapy and the emotional disorders*. New York: International Universities Press.

Beck, A.T., Emery, G., & Greenberg, R.L. (1985). *Anxiety disorders and phobias: a cognitive perspective*. New York: Basic Books.

Beck, A.T., Rush, A.J., Shaw, B.F., & Emery, G. (1979) *Cognitive therapy of depression*. New York: Guilford Press.

Beck, J. (1995). *Cognitive therapy: basics and beyond*. New York: Guilford.

Bennett-Levy, J., Butler, G., Fennell, M., Hackmann, A., Mueller, M., Rouf, K., & Westbrook, D. (2004). *Oxford guide to behavioural experiments in cognitive therapy*. Oxford: Oxford University Press.

Bentall, R. (2003). *Madness explained: Psychosis and human nature*. London: Penguin.

Bettleheim, B. (1984). *Freud and man's soul*. New York: Vintage Books.

Bieling, P.J. & Kuyken, W. (2003). Is cognitive case formulation science or science fiction? Clinical Psychology: *Science and Practice, 10*, 52–69.

Blenkiron, P. (2005). Stories and analogies in cognitive behaviour therapy: a clinical review. *Behavioural and Cognitive Psychotherapy, 33*, 45–59.

Borkovec, T.D., & Inz, J. (1990). The nature of worry in generalized anxiety disorder: a predominance of thought activity. *Behaviour Research and Therapy, 28*, 153–158.

Bosman, J. (1987). Persuasive effects of political metaphors. *Metaphor and Symbol, 2*, 97–113.

Bowdle, B.F., & Gentner, D. (2005). The career of metaphor. *Psychological Review, 112*, 193–216.

Brewin, C.R., & Holmes, E.A. (2003). Psychological theories of posttraumatic stress disorder. *Clinical Psychology Review, 23*(3), 339–376.

Brewin, C.R., Reynolds, M., & Tata, P. (1999). Autobiographical memory processes and the course of depression. *Journal of Abnormal Psychology, 108*, 511–517.

Burns, D.D. (1980). *Feeling good: the new mood therapy*. New York: Wm. Morrow and Co.

Burns, G.W. (2001). *101 healing stories: using metaphors in therapy*. Chichester, UK: Wiley.

Butler, G. (1998). Clinical formulation. In A.S. Bellack and M. Hersen (Eds) *Comprehensive Clinical Psychology*. New York: Pergammon Press.

Carey, T. A. (2006). *Method of levels: how to do psychotherapy without getting in the way.* Hayward, CA: Living Control Systems Publishing.

Carey, T.A., & Bourbon, W.T. (2006). Is countercontrol the key to understanding chronic behaviour problems? *Intervention in School & Clinic, 42*, 5–13.

Cartwright-Hatton, S., Roberts, C., Chitsabesan, P., Fothergill, C., & Harrington, R. (2004). Systematic review of the efficacy of cognitive behaviour therapies for childhood and adolescent anxiety disorders. *British Journal of Clinical Psychology, 43*, 421–436.

Clark, D.M. (1986). A cognitive approach to panic. *Behaviour Research and Therapy, 24*, 461–470.

Clark, D.M. (1999). Anxiety disorders: why they persist and how to treat them. *Behaviour Research and Therapy, 37*(S1), S5–S28.

Clark, D.M., & Teasdale, J.D. (1982). Diurnal variation in clinical depression and the accessibility of memories of positive and negative experiences. *Journal of Abnormal Psychology, 91*, 87–95.

Clark, D.M., & Wells, A. (1995). A cognitive model of social phobia. In R.G. Heimberg, M.R. Liebowitz, D.A. Hope, & F.R. Schneier (Eds.), *Social phobia: diagnosis, assessment, and treatment* (pp. 69–93). New York: Guilford Press.

Conway, M.A., & Pleydell-Pearce, C.W. (2000) The construction of autobiographical memories in the self-memory system. *Psychological Review, 107*, 261–288.

Dimidjian, S., Hollon, S.D., & Dobson, K.S. (2006). Randomized trial of behavioural activation, cognitive therapy, and antidepressant medication in the acute treatment of adults with major depression. *Journal of Consulting and Clinical Psychology, 74*, 658–670.

Dobson, K.S., Hollon, S.D., Dimidjian, S., Schmaling, K.B., Kohlenberg, R.J., Gallop, R.J., Rizvi, S.L., Gollan, J.K., Dunner, D.L., & Jacobson, N.S. (2008). Randomized trial of behavioural activation, cognitive therapy, and antidepressant medication in the prevention of relapse and recurrence in major depression. *Journal of Consulting and Clinical Psychology, 76*, 468–477.

Dugas, M.J. & Robichaud, M. (2006). *Cognitive-behavioural treatment for generalized anxiety disorder: From science to practice.* London: Routledge

Ehlers, A., & Breuer, P. (1992). Increased cardiac awareness in panic disorder. *Journal of Abnormal Psychology, 101*, 371–382.

Ehlers, A., & Clark, D.M. (2000). A cognitive model of posttraumatic stress disorder. *Behaviour Research and Therapy, 38*, 319–345.

Eysenck, H.J. (1979). The conditioning model of neurosis. *Behavioural and Brain Sciences, 2*, 155–166.

Fairburn, C.G., Cooper, Z., & Shafran, R. (2003). Cognitive behaviour therapy for eating disorders: 'transdiagnostic' theory and treatment. *Behaviour Research and Therapy, 41*, 509–528.

Fairburn, C.G., Shafran, R., & Cooper, Z. (1999). A cognitive-behavioural theory of anorexia nervosa. *Behaviour Research and Therapy, 37*, 1–14.

Feldman, J. & Narayanan, S. (2004). Embodied meaning in a neural theory of language. *Brain and language, 89*, 385–192.

Fennell, M. (1999). *Overcoming low self-esteem. A self-help guide using Cognitive Behavioural Techniques.* London: Robinson.

Field, A.P. (2006). Watch out for the beast: fear information and attentional bias in children. *Journal of Clinical Child and Adolescent Psychology, 35*(3), 431–439.

Flavell, J.H. (1979). Metacognition and cognitive monitoring: A new era of cognitive developmental inquiry. *American Psychologist, 34,* 906–s911.

Freeman, D., & Garety, P.A. (2004). Bats among birds. *The Psychologist, 17,* 642–645.

Freeston, M.H., Rheaume, J., Letarte, H., Dugas, M.J. & Ladouceur, R. (1994). Why do people worry? *Personality and Individual Differences, 17,* 791–802.

Garety, P., Kuipers, E., Fowler, D., Freeman, D., & Bebbington, P.E. (2001). A cognitive model of the positive symptoms of psychosis. *Psychological Medicine, 31,* 189–195.

Gibbs, R.W. (2003). Embodied experience and linguistic meaning. *Brain and Language, 84,* 1–15.

Gibran, K. (1992). *The prophet.* London: Penguin.

Gilbert, P. (1998). What is shame? Some core issues and controversies. In P. Gilbert & B. Andrews (Eds). *Shame: Interpersonal behaviour, psychopathology, and culture.* Oxford: Oxford University Press.

Gilbert, P., & Irons, C. (2004). Pilot exploration of the use of compassionate images in a group of self-critical people. *Memory, 12,* 507–516.

Gillan, D.J., Premack, D., & Woodruff, G. (1981). Reasoning in the chimpanzee: I. Analogical reasoning. *Journal of Experimental Psychology: Animal Behaviour Processes, 7,* 1–17.

Glucksberg, S. (2008). How metaphors create categories - quickly. In R.W. Gibbs (Ed.) *The Cambridge handbook of metaphor and thought.* Cambridge: Cambridge University Press.

Gordon, D.C. (1978). *Therapeutic metaphors: helping others through the looking glass.* Cupertino, CF: Meta Publications.

Griffin, J., & Tyrrell, I. (2006). *Dreaming reality: How dreaming keeps us sane, or can drive us mad.* Sussex, UK: HG Publishing.

Haidt, J. (2006). *The happiness hypothesis.* New York: Basic Books.

Harvey, A.G., Watkins, E.R., Mansell, W., & Shafran, R. (2004). *Cognitive behavioural processes across psychological disorders: A transdiagnostic approach to research and treatment.* Oxford: Oxford University Press.

Hassin, R.R., Uleman, J.S., & Bargh, J.A. (2005). *The new unconscious.* New York: Oxford University Press.

Hayes, S.C. (2004). Acceptance and Commitment Therapy and the new behaviour therapies: Mindfulness, acceptance, and relationship. In S.C. Hayes, V.M. Follette, & M.M. Linehan (Eds.), *Mindfulness and acceptance: Expanding the cognitive-behavioural tradition* (pp. 1–29). New York: Guilford Press.

Hayes, S.C., Barnes-Holmes, D., & Roche, B. (2001). *Relational frame theory: A post-Skinnerian account of human language and cognition.* New York: Plenum Press.

Hayes, S.C., & Smith, S. (2005). *Get out of your mind and into your life.* Oakland, CA: New Harbinger.

Hayes, S.C., Strosahl, K.D., & Wilson, K.G. (1999). *Acceptance and commitment therapy. An experiential approach to behaviour change.* New York: Guilford.

Hersen, M., & Barlow, D.H. (1976). *Single case experimental designs: strategies for studying behaviour change.* New York: Pergamon.

Jones, S.H. (2001). Circadian rhythms, multilevel models of emotion and bipolar disorder: An initial step towards integration? *Clinical Psychology Review, 21,* 1193–1209.

Jung, C.G. (1964). *Man and his symbols.* Mass Market Paperback. London: Aldus Books.

Kopp, R.R. (1995). *Metaphor therapy: Using client-generated metaphors in psychotherapy.* New York: Brunner-Mazel.

Kövecses, Z. (2000). *Metaphor and emotion: language, culture, and body in human feeling.* Cambridge: Cambridge University Press.

Kövecses, Z. (2002). *Metaphor: A practical introduction.* New York: Oxford University Press.

Kubany, E.S. (1998). Cognitive therapy for trauma-related guilt. In Follette, V.M., Ruzek, J.I., Abueg, F.R. (Eds) *Cognitive-behavioural therapies for trauma.* New York: Guilford Press.

Lakoff, G., & Johnson, M. (1980). *Metaphors we live by.* Chicago, IL: University of Chicago Press.

Lakoff, G., & Kovecses, Z. (1987). The cognitive model of anger inherent in American English. In D.C. Holland & N. Quinn (Eds). *Cultural models in language and thought, Chapter 8.* Cambridge: Cambridge University Press.

Lankton, C.H., & Lankton, S.R. (1989). *Tales of enchantment: goal-oriented metaphors for adults and children in therapy.* New York: Brunner-Mazel.

Lee, D.A. (2005). The perfect nurturer: A model to develop a compassaionate mind within the context of cognitive therapy. In P. Gilbert (Ed.). *Compassion: Conceptualisations, research and use in psychotherapy.* London: Brunner-Routledge.

Lidz, T. (1973) *The origin and treatment of schizophrenic disorders.* New York: Basic Books.

Locke, J. (1979). In P.H. Nidditch (Ed.). *An essay concerning human understanding.* New York: Oxford University Press.

Lopez, C., Tchanturia, K., Stahl, D., Booth, R., Holliday, J., & Treasure, J. (2008). An examination of the concept of central coherence in women with anorexia nervosa. *International Journal of Eating Disorders, 41,* 143–152.

Lule, J. (2004). War and its metaphors: news language and the prelude to war in Iraq, 2003. *Journalism Studies, 5,* 179–191.

Mansell, W. (2000). Conscious appraisal and the modification of automatic processes in anxiety. *Behavioural and Cognitive Psychotherapy, 28,* 99–120.

Mansell, W. (2005). Control theory and psychopathology. An integrative approach. *Psychology and Psychotherapy: Theory Research and Practice, 78,* 141–178.

Mansell, W. (2007). *Coping with fears and phobias: a step–by-step guide to understanding and facing your anxieties.* Oxford: OneWorld Press.

Mansell, W. (2008a). The seven Cs of CBT: A consideration of the future challenges for cognitive behavioural therapy. *Behavioural and Cognitive Psychotherapy, 36,* 641–649.

Mansell, W. (2008b). What is CBT *really* and how can we enhance the impact of effective psychotherapies such as CBT? In R. House & D. Loewenthal (Eds.), *Against and for CBT: Towards a constructive dialogue.* Ross-on-Wye, UK: PCCS Publications Ltd.

Mansell, W., & Hodson, S. (2009). Imagery and memories of the social self in people with bipolar disorders: empirical evidence, phenomenology, theory and therapy. In L. Stopa (Ed.), *Imagery and the threatened self: Perspectives on mental imagery in cognitive therapy*. Oxford: Routledge.

Mansell, W., & Lam, D. (2004). A preliminary study of autobiographical memory in remitted bipolar disorder and the role of imagery in memory specificity. *Memory, 12,* 437–446.

Mansell, W., Morrison, A.P., Reid, G., Lowens, I., & Tai, S. (2007). The interpretation of and responses to changes in internal states: an integrative cognitive model of mood swings and bipolar disorder. *Behavioural and Cognitive Psychotherapy, 35,* 515–539.

Mansell, W., & Pedley (2008). The ascent into mania: a review of psychological processes associated with manic symptoms. *Clinical Psychology Review, 28,* 494–520.

Mansell, W., Scott, J., & Colom, F. (2005). The nature and treatment of bipolar depression: Implications for psychological investigation. *Clinical Psychology Review, 25,* 1076–1100.

McCurry, S.M. & Hayes, S.C. (1992). Clinical and experimental perspectives on metaphorical talk. *Clinical Psychology Review, 12,* 763–785.

McGlone, M.S. (2007). What is the explanatory value of a conceptual metaphor? *Language and Communication, 27,* 109–126.

McMullen, L.M. (2008). Putting it in context: metaphor and psychotherapy. In R.W. Gibbs (Ed.) *The Cambridge handbook of metaphor and thought*. Cambridge: Cambridge University Press.

Meares, K., & Freeston, M. (2008). *Overcoming worry. A self-help guide using cognitive behavioural techniques*. London: Robinson.

Merwin, W.S. (1968). *Selected translations 1948–1968*. New York: Atheneum.

Miller, W.R., & Rollnick, S. (2002). *Motivational interviewing: Preparing people for change. 2nd Ed.* New York: Guilford.

Minsky, M. (1987). *The society of mind*. New York: Simon & Schuster.

Morrison, A.P. (2001). The interpretation of intrusions in psychosis: An integrative cognitive approach to hallucinations and delusions. *Behavioural and Cognitive Psychotherapy, 29,* 257–276.

Morrison, A.P., Beck, A.T., Glentworth, D., Dunn, H., Reid, G.S., Larkin, W., & Williams, S. (2002). Imagery and psychotic symptoms: a preliminary investigation. *Behaviour Research and Therapy, 40,* 1053–1062.

Muran, J.C., & DiGiuseppe, R.A. (1990). Towards a cognitive formulation of metaphor use in psychotherapy. *Clinical Psychology Review, 10,* 69–85.

Nehaniv, C. (1999). *Computation for metaphors, analogy, and agents: Lecture Notes in Computer Science, 1562*. London: Springer.

Nolen-Hoeksema, S. (1991). Responses to depression and their effects on the duration of depressive episodes. *Journal of Abnormal Psychology, 100,* 569–582.

Oden, D.L., Thompson, R.K.R., and Premack, D. (2001). Can an ape reason analogically? In D. Gentner, K.J. Holyoak, & B.N. Kokinov, (Eds.), *The analogical mind: Perspectives from cognitive science*. Cambridge, MA: MIT Press (chap. 14).

Ortony, A. (Ed.) (1993). *Metaphor and thought* (2nd Ed.). New York: Cambridge University Press.

Otto, M. (2000) Stories and metaphors in cognitive-behaviour therapy. *Cognitive and Behavioural Practice, 7,* 166–172.

Padesky, C.A. (1990). Schema as self-prejudice. *International Cognitive Therapy Newsletter,* *6,* 6–7.

Padesky, C.A. (1994). Schema change processes in cognitive thearpy. *Clinical Psychology and Psychotherapy, 1,* 267–278.

Paris, R. (2002). Kosovo and the metaphor war. *Political Science Quarterly, 117,* 423–450.

Persons, J.B. & Tompkins, M.A. (2007). Cognitive-behavioural case formulation. In T.D. Eells (Ed) *Handbook of psychotherapy case formulation, 2nd Ed.* New York: Guilford.

Powers, W.T. (1973, 2005). *Behaviour: the control of perception.* New Canaan, CT: Benchmark Publications.

Proudfoot, J., Swain, S., Widmer, S., Watkins, E., Goldberg, D., Marks, I., Mann, A., & Gray, J.A. (2003). The development and beta-test of a computer-therapy program for anxiety and depression: Hurdles and preliminary outcomes. *Computers in Human Behaviour, 19,* 277–289.

Rachman, S.J., de Silva, P., & Roper, G. (1976). The spontaneous decay of compulsive urges. *Behaviour Research and Therapy, 14,* 445–453.

Rapee, R., & Heimberg, R. (1997). A cognitive behavioural model of anxiety in social phobia. *Behaviour Research and Therapy, 35,* 741–756.

Richards, I.A. (1936). *The Philosophy of rhetoric.* New York: Oxford University Press.

Rosen, S. (1982) (Ed) *My voice will go with you: The teaching tales of Milton H. Erickson, M.D.* New York: W.W. Norton.

Rowe, D. (2003). *Depression. The way out of your prison* (3rd ed.). Hove: Brunner-Routledge.

Salkovskis, P.M. (1985). Obsessional-compulsive problems: A cognitive-behavioural analysis. *Behaviour Research and Therapy, 25,* 571–583.

Salkovskis, P.M. (1988). Phenomenology, assessment and the cognitive model of panic. In S.J. Rachman & J. Maser (Eds). *Panic: Psychological perspectives.* Hillsdale, NJ: Erlbaum.

Salkovskis, P.M. (1996). The cognitive approach to anxiety: threat beliefs, safety-seeking behaviour, and the special case of health anxiety and obsessions. In P. M. Salkovskis (Ed.), *Frontiers of cognitive therapy* (pp. 48–74). New York: Guilford Press.

Salkovskis, P.M. (2002). Empirically grounded clinical interventions: Cognitive-behavioural therapy progresses through a multi-dimensional approach to clinical science. *Behavioural and Cognitive Psychotherapy, 30,* 3–9.

Salkovskis, P.M., & Campbell, P. (1994). Thought suppression induces intrusion in naturally occurring negative thoughts. *Behaviour Research and Therapy, 32,* 1–8.

Salkovskis, P.M., Clark, D.M., Hackmann, A., Wells, A., & Gelder, M.G. (1999). An experimental investigation of the role of safety-seeking behaviours in the maintenance of panic disorder with agoraphobia. *Behaviour Research and Therapy, 37,* 559–574.

Sanders, M.R. (1999). Triple P-positive parenting program: Towards an empirically validated multilevel parenting and family support strategy for the prevention of behaviour and emotional problems in children. *Clinical Child and Family Psychology Review, 2*(2), 71–90.

Schmidt, U., Bone, G., Hems, S., Lessem, J. & Treasure, J. (2002). Structured therapeutic writing tasks as an adjunct to treatment in eating disorders. *European Eating Disorders Review, 10,* 299–315.

Seal, K., Mansell, W., & Mannion, H. (2008). What lies between hypomania and bipolar disorder? A qualitative analysis of twelve non-treatment-seeking people with a history of hypomanic experiences and no history of major depression. *Psychology and Psychotherapy: Theory, Research and Practice, 81*, 33–53.

Segal, Z., Williams, J.M.G., & Teasdale, J.D. (2002). *Mindfulness-based cognitive therapy for depression.* New York: Guilford Press.

Seligman, M.E.P. (1988). Competing theories of panic. In S. Rachman & J.D. Maser (Eds) *Panic: Psychological perspectives.* Hillsdale, NJ: Erlbaum.

Selfridge, O.G. (1959). Pandemonium: A paradigm for learning. In D.V. Blake and A.M. Uttley (Eds.), *Proceedings of the Symposium on Mechanisation of Thought Processes,* pp. 511–529.

Smucker, M.R., & Dancu, C.V. (1999). *Cognitive-behavioural treatment for adult survivors of childhood trauma: Imagery rescripting and reprocessing.* Northvale, NJ: Jason Aronson.

Soskice, J.M. (1987). *Metaphor and religious language.* Oxford: Clarendon Press.

Stein, G. (1947). *Four in America.* New Haven: Yale University Press.

Stott, R. (2007). When head and heart do not agree: a theoretical and clinical analysis of rational-emotional dissociation (RED) in cognitive therapy. *Journal of Cognitive Psychotherapy, 21*, 37–50.

Szasz, T. (1976) *Schizophrenia: The sacred symbol of psychiatry.* New York: Basic Books.

Tang, T.Z., & DeRubeis, R.J. (1999). Sudden gains and critical sessions in cognitive-behavioural therapy for depression. *Journal of Consulting and Clinical Psychology, 67*(6), 894–904.

Teasdale, J.D. (1993). Emotion and two kinds of meaning: Cognitive therapy and applied cognitive science. *Behaviour Research and Therapy, 31*, 339–354.

Teasdale, J., & Barnard, P. (1993). *Affect, cognition and change.* Hove, UK: Lawrence Erlbaum Associates.

Tolton, J.C. (2006). Rogue psychotic mindset—the seat of delusive misconception? *Behavioural and Cognitive Psychotherapy, 34*, 487–490.

Treasure, J., & Schmidt, U. (2006). Anorexia nervosa: valued and visible. A cognitive-interpersonal maintenance model and its implications for research and practice. *British Journal of Clinical Psychology, 45*, 343–366.

Treasure, J., & Schmidt, U. (2007). The Maudsley model individual treatment manual for anorexia nervosa. Unpublished treatment manual.

Trinder, H. & Salkovskis, P.M. (1994). Personally relevant intrusions outside the laboratory: long-term suppression increases intrusion. *Behaviour Research and Therapy, 32*, 833–842.

Waller, G., Cordery, H., Corstorphine, E., Hinrichsen, H., Lawson, R., Mountford, V., & Russell, K. (2007). *Cognitive-behavioural therapy for the eating disorders: A comprehensive treatment guide.* Cambridge, UK: Cambridge University Press.

Watkins, E.R. (2008). Constructive and unconstructive repetitive thought. *Psychological Bulletin, 134*, 163–206.

Watkins, E., & Baracaia, S. (2002). Rumination and social problem solving in depression. *Behaviour Research and Therapy, 40*, 1179–1189.

Webster-Stratton, C., Reid, M., & Hammond, M. (2004). Treating children with early-onset conduct problems: intervention outcomes for parent, child, and teacher training. *Journal of Clinical Child and Adolescent Psychology, 33*(1), 105–124.

Wedding, D., Boyd, M.A., & Niemiec, R.M. (2005). *Movies and mental illness: Using films to understand psychopathology.* Cambridge, MA: Hogrefe & Huber.

Weertman, A., & Arntz, A. (2007). Effectiveness of treatment of childhood memories in cognitive therapy for personality disorders: A controlled study contrasting methods focusing on the present and methods focusing on childhood memories. *Behaviour Research and Therapy, 45,* 2133–2143.

Wegner, D.M., & Zanakos, S. (1994). Chronic thought suppression. *Journal of Personality, 62,* 615–640.

Wells, A. (1997). *Cognitive therapy of anxiety disorders: A practical guide.* Bognor Regis, UK: Wiley-Blackwell.

Wells, A. (2000). *Emotional disorders and metacognition: Innovative cognitive therapy.* Chichester, UK: Wiley.

Wells, A. (2007). The attentional training technique: Theory, effects and a metacognitive hypothesis on auditory hallucinations. *Cognitive and Behavioural Practice, 14,* 134–138.

Wheatley, J., Brewin, C.R., Patel, T., Hackmann, A., Wells, A., Fisher, P. & Myers, S. (2007). "I'll believe it when I can see it": Imagery rescripting of intrusive sensory memories in depression. *Journal of Behaviour Therapy and Experimental Psychiatry, 38,* 371–385.

Williams, J.M.G., Teasdale, J.D., Segal, Z., & Kabat-Zinn, J. (2007). *The mindful way through depression.* New York: Guilford Press.

Wolff, G., & Serpell, L. (1998). A cognitive model and treatment strategies for anorexia nervosa. In H. Hoek, J. Treasure, & M. Katzman (Eds,), *Neurobiology in the treatment of eating disorders.* Chichester: Wiley.

Wolfe, K.K., & Wolfe, G.K. (1976). Metaphors of madness: Popular psychological narratives. *The Journal of Popular Culture, 9,* 895–907.

Young, J.E., Klosko, J.S., & Weishaar, M.E. (2003). *Schema therapy: A practitioner's guide.* New York: Guilford Press.

Zibart, E. *When the healer and patient are one.* Interview with Lauren Slater. Retrieved on June 6, 2008 from http://www.bookpage.com/9602bp/nonfiction/welcometomycountry.html.

Index

Abuse, 205
Acceptance and commitment therapy
     (ACT), 13, 90
     cognitive fusion, 61
Activation stage of metaphor use, 21
Activity
     as medicine, 119
     scheduling, 118
Affective avoidance, 136
All or nothing thinking, 113
All the world's a stage, 5
Amygdala
     as guard dog, 153
     and hippocampus, 153
Anger, 210
     as hot fluid in container, 12
Anorexia, 191
Anxiety, 127
     anxious child's radar, 224
     disorder specific factors, 140
     facing your fears, 136
     factors across disorders, 132
     maintenance of, 130
     selective attention, 130
     threat appraisal, 128
Architect and Surveyor, 51
Argument as war, 12
Aristotle, 8
Ars poetica, 8
Assertiveness, 210
Assumptions as personal contracts, 111
Attention shifting in social phobia, 150
Automaticity, 79
Avoidance, 136

Bad cup metaphor, 13
Bad news radio, 94
Balancing emotions, 34
Ball of string metaphor, 65
Barrier metaphors
     affective avoidance, 136
     in bipolar disorder, 166
     isolation and depression, 111
Behaviour
     behavioural activation, 118
     behavioural avoidance, 136
     behavioural experiments, 52
Beliefs
     as the 'bottom line', 110
     as buttons being pressed, 110
     as hogging the airtime, 118

as needing road-testing, 118
Benzene ring, insight and discovery, 97
Bike stabilisers
     graded behaviours as, 139
     medication as, 70
Bipolar disorder, 159
     client's metaphors for internal states, 162
     as dangerous gift, 167
     Icarus story, 168
     as part of self, 105
     potholes and lampposts, 171
Black and white thinking, 113
Black hole, 59
Blame and responsibility, 216
Boat on rough sea, 166
Botox face, 224
Brain as camera, 59
Brand new shoes metaphor, 118
Break it down metaphor, 219
Breath of Fresh Air, 5
Bribe, taking a small, 148
Bridge building, 28, 33, 132
Broken leg metaphor, 1, 32
Brushing teeth metaphor, 55, 83
Bucket with hole, 175
Builder's apprentice metaphor, 16, 137, 141
Bulimia, 199
Bully
     giving in to, 63
     OCD as, 145
     separation of bullying and bullied, 122
Burglar metaphor, 58
Bursting into tears: fear of 'snapping', 42
Business consultant, therapist as, 53

CAKE metaphor, for causality, 216
Car crash metaphor, for responsibility, 217
Car Insurance, taking responsibility, 55
Case formulation, 40
CBT
     as 'The Borg', 69
     as family of therapies, 68
     as football, 50
     as surgery, 73
Changing gear, automaticity, 79
Child and iron metaphor, 213
Child who is afraid of dogs, 136
Churchill, Winston, 9
Client
     as explorer, 34
     as scientist, 52

as script writer, 183
client-generated metaphors, 45
Clinical art and clinical science, 48, 228
Clouds crossing sky, 95, 125
Coach, therapist as, 52
Cognitive avoidance, 136
Cognitive behavioural therapy, *see* CBT
Cognitive specificity
  burglar metaphor, 58
  dog mess story, 36, 37
Collaborative relationship, 50
Columbo, therapist as, 51
Compactness hypothesis, 15
Complex systems as plants, 12
Conceptual metaphor, 10
Conservation of mental energy, 121
Constructivism, 10
Continuum metaphor, 114
Control and resistance, 53
Control of thoughts, 92
Cross-cultural issues, 42

D for distinction, 58
Dark Cloud, 6
Dark glasses metaphor, 114
Dead metaphors, 16, 42
Death, 7
Deep-rooted Issues, 6
Depression
  as battle, 107
  as black dog, 105
  as darkness, 105
  as gargoyle, 122
  as gravitational pull, 105
  as weight, 106
Detective, therapist as, 51
Dichotomous thinking, 113
Digging a hole, in bipolar disorder, 164
Digging to get out of a hole
  counterproductive strategies, 132
  reassurance seeking, 39
  shovel and ladder, 62
  trying too hard, 145
  vicious cycles, 61
Distancing function, 29
Distorting lens, 5
Divided parts of the self, 87
Dog mess metaphor, 36, 44, 58
Double-edged sword, 97
Dragon in mountain, 220
Dreaming while awake, 177
Dress rehearsal, therapy as, 53
Driving on other side, 83

Eating disorders, 189
  acclimatisation on mountain, 193
  as addiction, 199
  airline pilot, 192

all eggs in one basket, 198
drops in reservoir, 194
as external entities, 196
food as medicine, 192
as friend and enemy, 198
gilded cage, 191
holding your breath, 195
itchy jumper, 196
keeping the car going, 192
little lives, little selves, 191
uninvited guest at party, 199
Elaboration stage of metaphor use, 23
Electrical voltage metaphor, 114
Elephant, mind as, 82
Elephants on the track metaphor, 138
Embodied cognition, 17
Emotions
  anger, 12, 37, 47, 210
  anxiety, 127
  emotional metaphors to engage, 28
  guilt, 212
  low mood, 105, 125, 160, 162, 164
  and metaphor, 14
  shame, 212
Empirically grounded clinical interventions, 229
Enacting metaphor, 28
Erickson and metaphor, 12
Escalator, 6
Eureka moment, 97
Expectancy biases, 88
Experiential avoidance: unexploded bomb
  metaphor, 109
Explorer, client as, 34
Extinction, 129

Fables, 7
Fairy stories, 7
False alarms and emergencies, 127
Family of therapies, CBT as, 68
Fault lines, 124
Fawlty Towers, 60
Feeding the tiger metaphor, 93
Ferris wheel thoughts, 120
Fierce dragon in hills, 96
Figurative language, 8
Filing cabinet, memory as, 85
Films, *see* Movies
Filter, lens, 59
Flexible foundations for strong buildings, 111
Flipsides of same coin, 164
Football, CBT as, 50
Foreign market metaphor, 43
Formulation, 40, 56
  how therapy works, 38
  as map, 40, 57

Gargoyle of depression, 122
Generalised anxiety disorder (GAD), 155

Ghosts from the past, 124
Gilded cage, 191
Giving birth, as emotional metaphor, 28
Glass box metaphor, 150
Glass half full, 58
Gloomy pair of spectacles, 14
Going to the Post Office, 52
Gollum and Smeagol, as voices in
    dialogue, 181
Graded behaviours
    as bike stabilisers, 140
    as scaffolding, 139
Grand canyon, tightrope over, 84
Grasping ideas, 22
Grooves in a track, 124
Guard dog, amygdala as, 153
Guilt, 212
Gun barrel effect, 135

Habituation, 129
Head versus heart, 36, 51
Health anxiety, 148
Health vs illness, taking responsibility, 55
Hitting rock bottom, 97
Homework
    as exercise, 67
    as skill learning, 67
How the Mind Works, 79
Huddled into a ball, 164
Humour, 44, 139

Icarus, 168
Imagery, 19, 20, 22, 24, 45, 89, 123, 177, 205
Independence versus dependence, 203
Inertia and effort, 67
Inexpressibility hypothesis, 15
Infected wound metaphor, 148
Inner conflict, 96
Insight, 97
Insurance metaphor, 146
Intellectual versus emotional belief, 86
Interacting cognitive subsystems (ICS), 24
Interpersonal difficulties, 201
Iron Curtain, 9
Isolation and withdrawal, 111
Itching a rash, 63

Jigsaw metaphor, 152
Journey metaphors
    course of therapy as journey, 64
    unfolding processes, 63
Judo metaphor, 206

Kick-starting system, 119
King, Martin Luther, 9
Kopp, Richard: metaphor therapy, 14

Lakoff and Johnson, 10

Learning
    to cycle, 194
    habituation and extinction, 129
    learning theory in anxiety, 127
Leaves, NATs as, 86
Lens
    distorting lens, 5
    filter, 59, 114
Life is a journey, 11
Lightbulb, insight, 97
Limbic kid metaphor, 154
Little lives, little selves, 191
Locke, John, 9
Looking for trouble, 133
Lurgy school game, 208

Managing company, 82
Marble in cone, 59
Medical analogies, 70
Medical examination, assessment as, 63
Medication as bike stabilisers, 70
Memory
    doing the talking, 124, 155
    influence of past memories, 123
    overfull cupboard, 15, 85, 151
Metacognition, 75, 89
Metaphor
    client-generated metaphors, 45
    conceptual metaphor, 10
    historical roots, 7
    in other therapies, 12
    interactive view, 10
    as manipulation, 9
    metaphoric cognition, 14
    selection of right metaphor, 41
    working model of use, 21
Mind
    as elephant, 82
    how the mind works, 79
    mind train, 95
    as an organisation, 53
    as train platform, 108
Mindfulness, 95, 124
Mnemonic function of metaphor, 16
Model of metaphor use, 20, 21
Mood
    as colour, 105
    gravitational metaphor, 105
    swings, 159
    as vertical position, 105
    as weight, 105
Mountains
    to climb, 63
    therapist as mountain guide, 64
Movies
    Adaptation, 89
    A Beautiful Mind, 89, 186
    Clockwise, 94

Donnie Darko, 186
The Fisher King, 186
Guess Who's Coming to Dinner, 203
Lord of the Rings, 179
Parenthood, 89
Ratatouille, 171
Shine, 171
The Simpsons, 99
Strictly Ballroom, 171
Moving On, 11
Musical instruments, practice and, 84
Myths, 7

Negative automatic thoughts, 85
Negotiation and guided discovery, 30

Obsessive-compulsive disorder (OCD),
    131, 144
  as an addiction, 145
  insurance metaphor, 146
Old woman and rug metaphor, 121
Organisation and coherence, 84
Oscar-winning performance, 244
Overfull cupboard, memory as, 15, 85, 151
Overgeneralisation, 114
Overheard phone conversation, 35
Oversized duvet, 15

Pact with the devil, 148
Panic disorder, 141
  expert on own symptoms, 143
  waking at baby noises, 143
  waking needing lavatory, 143
Parables, 7
Paranoia, *Lord of the Rings*, 179
Parents
  expectations of children, 201
  parental attachment, 204
  parenting hotspots, 222
  parenting pyramid, 218
Partner and best friend metaphor, 39
Passivity, 211
Perceptual Control Theory (PCT), 24, 53
Perceptual narrowing, 135
Perfect nurturer imagery, 123
Perfectionism, 113
Philosophy and metaphor, 8
Pink Elephant, 60
Poetry, 8
  use of, 100
Political metaphor, 9
Post Office, going to, 52
Post Traumatic Stress Disorder, *see* PTSD
Practice, importance of, 84
Pregnant women, selective attention, 134
Prejudice metaphor, 115
Pressure Cooker, 176, 211
Probability and awfulness, 128

Problems as physical obstructions, 6
Promised land, 9
Psychoanalysis and metaphor, 13
Psychological problem as medical condition, 70
Psychosis, 173
  as a metaphor, 176
  as dream state, 177
  as illness, 174
  metacognitive approaches, 179
  narratives in popular culture, 185
  narrow path metaphor, 185
  rogue mindset, 100
  synesthesia, 181
PTSD, 151
  amygdala and hippocampus, 156
  guard dog, 153
  jigsaw metaphor, 152
  as life robber, 155
  overfull cupboard, 15, 85, 151
  oversensitive alarm, 154
Push-starting car metaphor, 119

Quicksand metaphor, 93, 125

Radar operators, 135
Radio station, tuning to, 150
Rail inspector metaphor, 109
Rational-emotional dissociation (RED), 87
Reassurance, 39
Recurrent thinking, 88, 92
Reframe stage of metaphor use, 23
Resilience, and flexibility, 111
Resistance and control, 53
Responsibility for change, 54
  car insurance metaphor, 55
  health vs illness, 55
Rewriting the rulebook, 110
Rigid rules, and earthquakes, 111
Rivers of blood, 10
Road testing beliefs, 118
Rock and a hard place, 97
Rocking the boat, 147
Role play, use of, 30
Roots, core beliefs as, 86
Rose is a rose is a rose, 8
Rules
  and beliefs, 110
  breaking, 150
  as tools for a job, 111
Rumination, 88, 119
Running marathon, 84

Safety-seeking behaviours, 130, 131, 135, 137
  builder's apprentice, 137
  elephants on the track, 137
  personification, 139
Scaffolding metaphor, 139
Schemas, 114

fighting for survival, 116
Scientist, client as, 52
Script metaphor, 94
See-saw metaphor, 212
Selective attention, 132
  client as expert, 134
  cocktail party, 181
  coming across new word, 134
  new purchases, 134
  pregnant women, 134
  as spotlight, 88
Selective memory, 88
Selective processing, 88
Self
  as dynamic entity, 68
  self-criticism, 122
Shame, 212
Sick child metaphor, 217
Simpsons, The, 99
Skating on thin ice, 136
Skill learning metaphor, for 'grey-scale
  thinking', 114
Snail without shell, as vulnerability, 206
Snakes, benzene dream, 97
Snapping, 6
  in anxiety, 143
  fear of, 42
Snowball, 105
Social network, as spider's web, 209
Social phobia, 149
  broadening the bandwidth, 150
  out of your head and into the world, 150
  self as glass box, 150
  tuning into radio station, 150
Spaghetti thoughts, 76, 120
Spider's web, 209
Spoiling the joke: use of humour, 44
Sporting performance, and practice, 84
Stress
  as bucket with hole, 175
  as a burden, 6
  special forces training, 143
  training for sporting events, 144
Surfing the waves, 124
Swan gliding upstream, 31
Swimming the Channel, 84
Sword of truth, 10
Synesthesia metaphor, 181
Synthesis stage of metaphor use, 22

Tabula Rasa, 9
Tea making, automaticity, 79
Teacher training programmes, 123
Tennis balls of worry, 94
Theoretical model of metaphor use, 20, 21
Theories as buildings, 11
Therapeutic relationship, 50

Therapist
  as biographer, 56
  as business consultant, 53
  as coach, 52
  as detective, 51
  as mountain guide, 64
  as project supervisor, 52
  as witness, 54
Therapy, as dress rehearsal, 56
Thoughts
  as clouds, 95
  thought suppression, 109, 131
Threat perception equation, 128
Time as motion, 12
Tolton, J.M., 179
Tool kit metaphor, 202
Tools for a job, rules as, 111
Traffic lights metaphor
  rituals in OCD, 144
  for rule-governed behaviour, 110
Train platform, mind as, 108
Trainee air-traffic controller, 128
Trapped, 5
Tug of war with monster, 93
Two experts in room, 50
  architect and surveyor, 51
Two minds, being in, 97
Typing a letter, 79

Verbal and imaginal cognition, 19
Vicious cycles, 61
Vicious flower, 132, 148
Vividness hypothesis, 15

War on terror, 10
Warrior princess, 164
Washing machine metaphor, 218
Waves, as mood, 166
Way through, 6
Weed thoughts, 118
Weights, balancing priorities, 97
Whirlpool, 59
White bear effect, 92
Wise tales, 7
Wittgenstein's family resemblances, 69
Wizard of Oz, 205
Worry
  allergy metaphor, 156
  seeds of doubt, 156
  tennis balls of worry, 94
  traffic flow metaphor, 156
  whirlwind, 156

Yes buts..., 116

Zipper mouth, 224
Zooming in, 135